Galley Girls

IN THE CITY

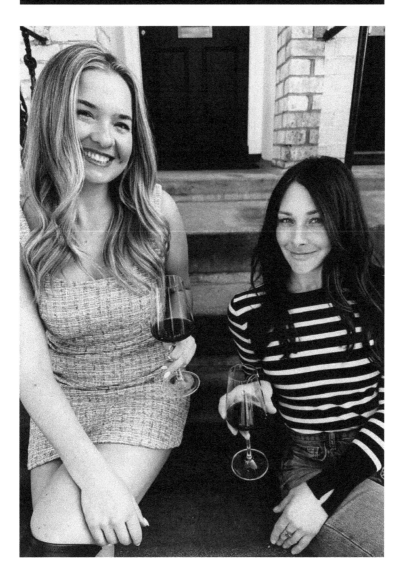

Daisy Kelliher & Bryony Johnson

GALLEY GIRLS - IN THE CITY

Published by Fisher King Publishing

fisherkingpublishing.co.uk

Three things
are needed
for a
good life...

Good friends
Good songs
and
Good food.

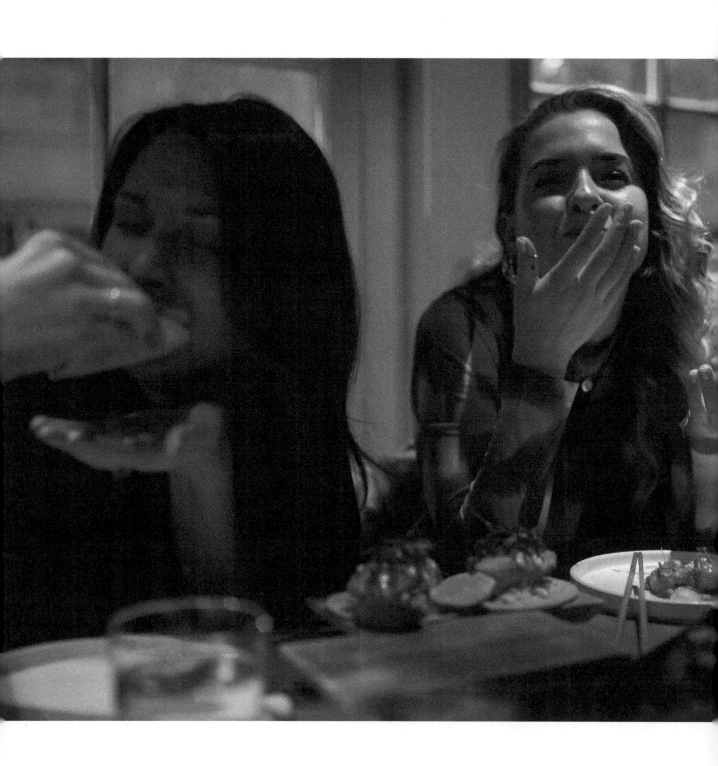

Hello... from the Galley Girls!

Daisy and Bryony's 'love affair' starts in Antigua 2017... Daisy was a stewardess on a private sailing yacht that was without a chef, a dangerous situation to be in with hungry guests and crew. In bounces Bryony, with all her flair and enthusiasm to be the galley ninja. The ladies' bonded instantly; two young females, foot-loose and fancy-free.

Their friendship grew as they discovered their mutual love of food, margaritas and rocking the dance floor. They shared the drive to work hard and, on rare moments ashore, play even harder. A great crew is built around the pairing of the chef and chief stewardess, and Bryony and Daisy brought the energy to the boat. You could even say that's where 'Daisy does drama started.'

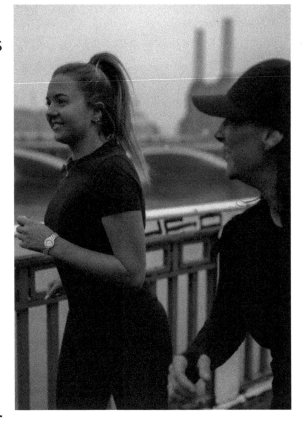

This created a friendship full of giggles and infectious laughter which resonated throughout the boat; boom, you have the birth of the Galley Girls!

Fast forward to winter 2021, Bryony and Daisy were working in the Caribbean. Europe was in lockdown and locally there were strict covid restrictions. The future was fragile and uncertain. Free days were spent hiking to remote beaches and through rainforests while trying to decipher what their futures held. Little did they know that they would both end up in London at the same time, and just around the corner from each other.

Countless hours were spent cooking, eating and sampling the local rum (which is where all the best ideas come from!). They wanted to share Bryony's expertise in nutrition and Daisy's passion for food, to create recipes that make your mouth water but were still nutritional and nourishing. The Galley Girls went from a small kitchen on a boat to developing a cookbook that anyone with a desire for guilt-free food can enjoy! xx

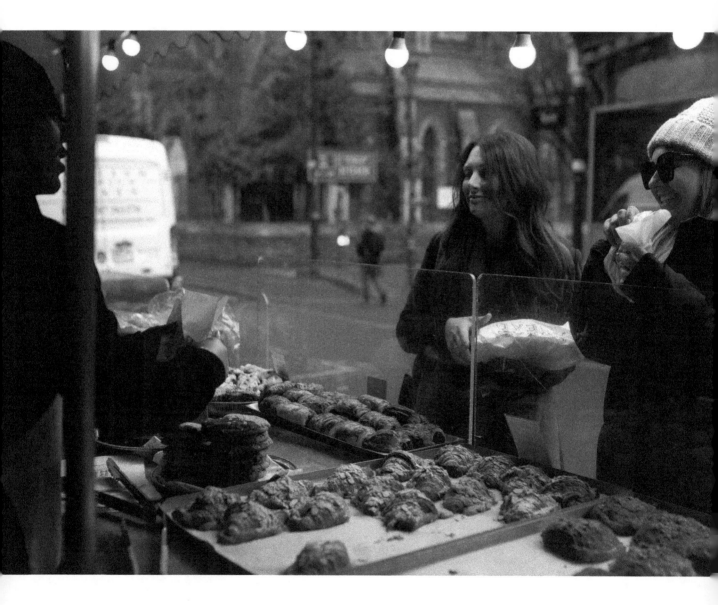

Bryony Johnson & Daisy Kelliher

CONTENTS

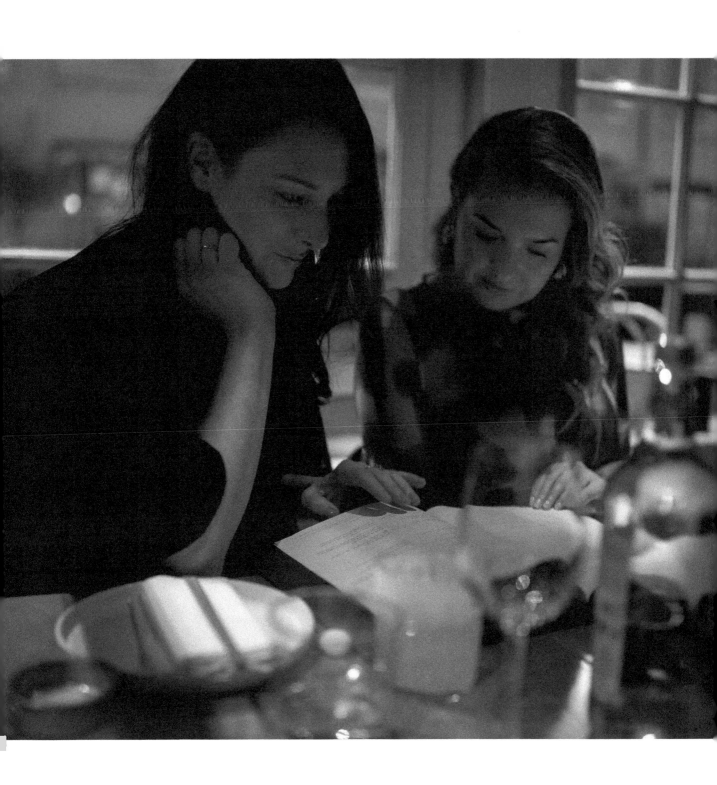

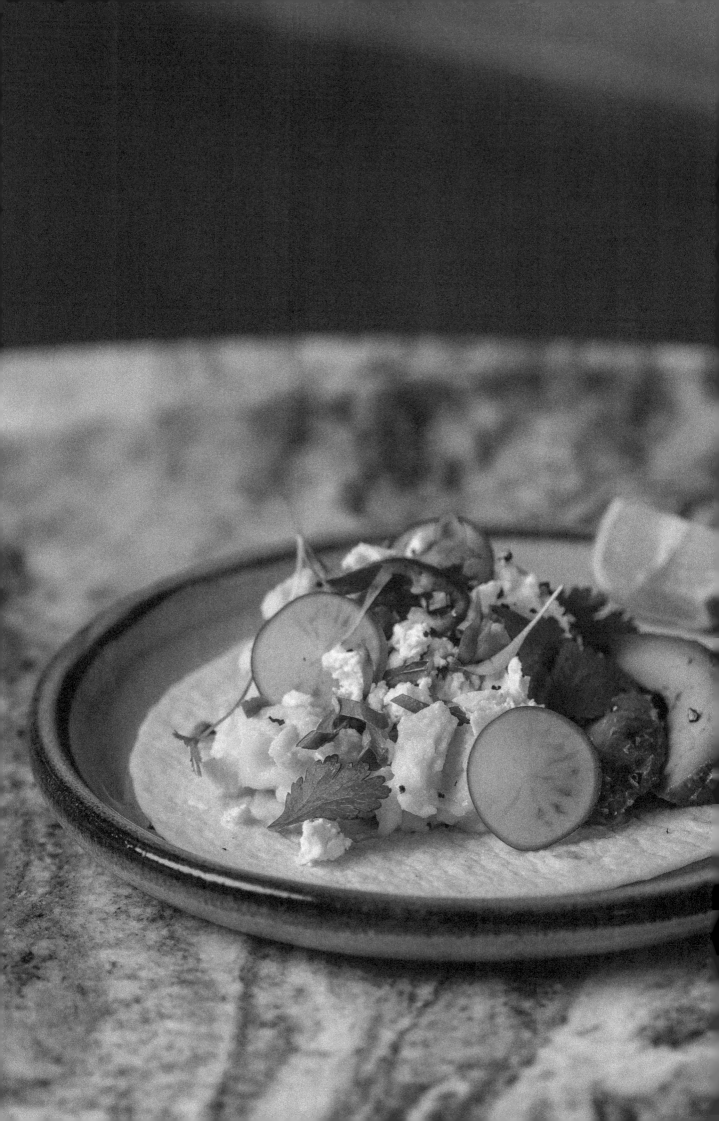

Breakfast Tacos

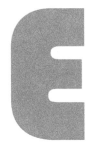njoy an eggcellant start to your day (apologies for that rubbish joke) with these breakfast tacos. They are so easy and versatile, can be made vegan by using scrambled tofu if eggs are not your thing! Such a healthy and delicious way to start your day.

Ingredients

Serves 4

8 corn tortillas

2 small ripe avocados

8 eggs / for vegans scrambled tofu

1 bunch scallions / spring onions

1 bunch fresh cilantro / coriander

1 jar of jalapenos

4oz / 100g feta or plant based alterative

4 radishes, sliced

2 limes

1 tbsp butter or olive oil

Salt and pepper

Method

1. In a small blender (I'm obsessed with my Nutribullet, I use it so much I think it's going to go on strike) roughly blend half the jar of jalapenos, with half a bunch of fresh coriander, juice of 1 lime and a pinch of salt. You are looking for a salsa like texture. Set aside.

2. On a chopping board, slice your radish, slice your avocado, cut your spring onions into 1cm rings. Season your radish, avocado and onions with salt and pepper and a little squeeze of lime. Roughly chop your coriander.

3. In a medium bowl crack your eggs, whisk them (also check you haven't got any sneaky bits of eggshell in there).

4. In a frying pan on a medium to low heat gently melt 1tbsp butter or oil, add your eggs, gently stir until you have lovely creamy scrambled eggs cooked to your liking. Take off the heat and season with salt and pepper.

5. Take your tortillas and divide onto your plates. Put your avocado, eggs, onions, radish on to your tortillas. Sprinkle feta over your eggs and then drizzle with that yummy spicy jalapeno, cilantro salsa. Scatter with a few more coriander leaves and these breakfast tacos are ready to get your mouth around, go for it!

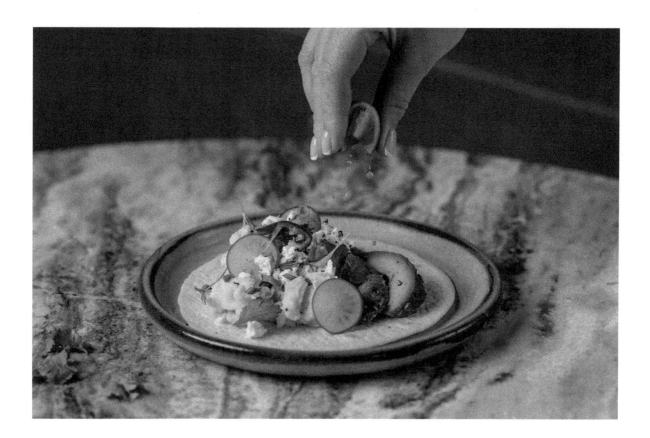

Bryony Johnson & Daisy Kelliher

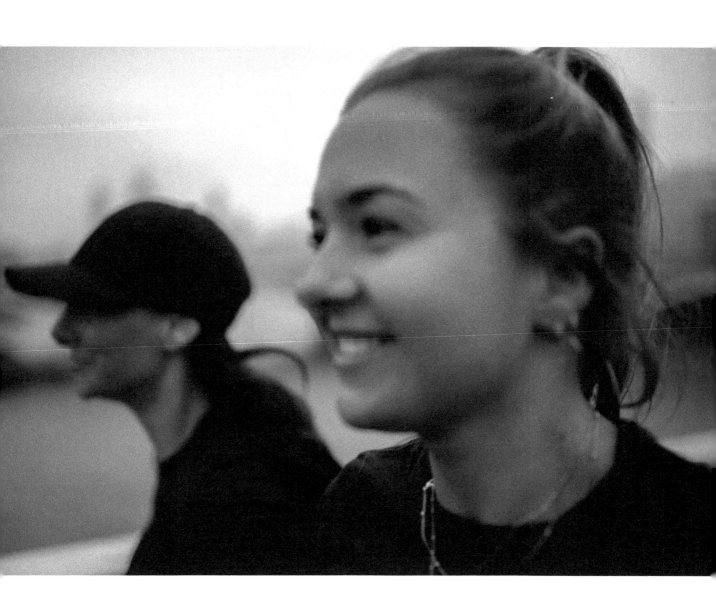

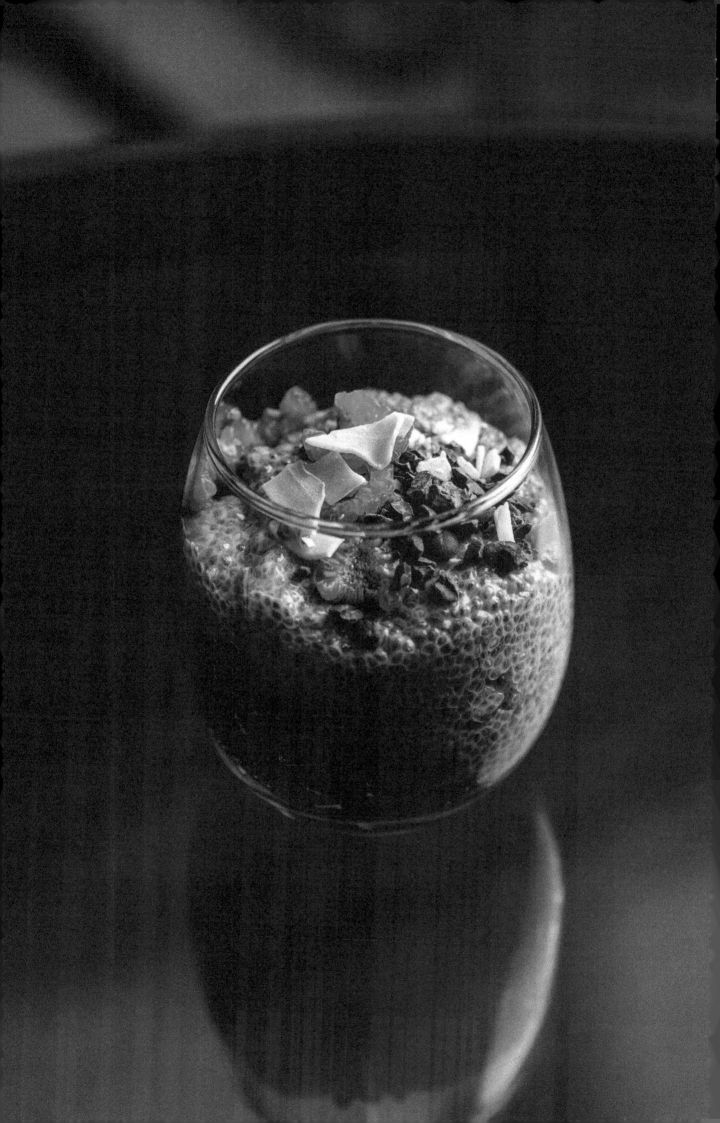

PB & Raspberry Chia Pudding

Top tip, make this breakfast the night before so it is ready to rock in the morning! It takes less than five minutes to prep. Let's go! You can add any topping you like Raspberries, peanut butter and toasted coconut is one of our favourites. For a more tropical taste, try mango and passion fruit with some cocoa nibs, delish! Full of calcium, antioxidants and fibre, your gut will love you!

Ingredients
Serves 2

5 tbsp chia seeds

1 ½ cups of coconut milk, or your preferred milk

1 tbsp of maple syrup

2 tbsp of your favourite nut butter

2 cups of raspberries

1 tsp of pure vanilla bean paste (optional)

Pinch of salt

Raspberries, blueberries, cocoa nibs and toasted coconut flakes optional toppings to jazz up your morning!

Method

1. In a medium bowl, combined the chia seeds, milk and stir well to avoid any chucks. Add the maple, vanilla bean and pinch of salt and mix everything well. Cover your bowl and switch into an airtight container. Leave in the fridge over night or for 1 hour in the fridge.

2. When you are ready to eat your chia pudding mash up your

raspberries with a fork in a bowl. Then get your small glasses layer up with some pureed raspberry then chia pudding. Add your nut butter and desired toppings and enjoy your delicious breakfast.

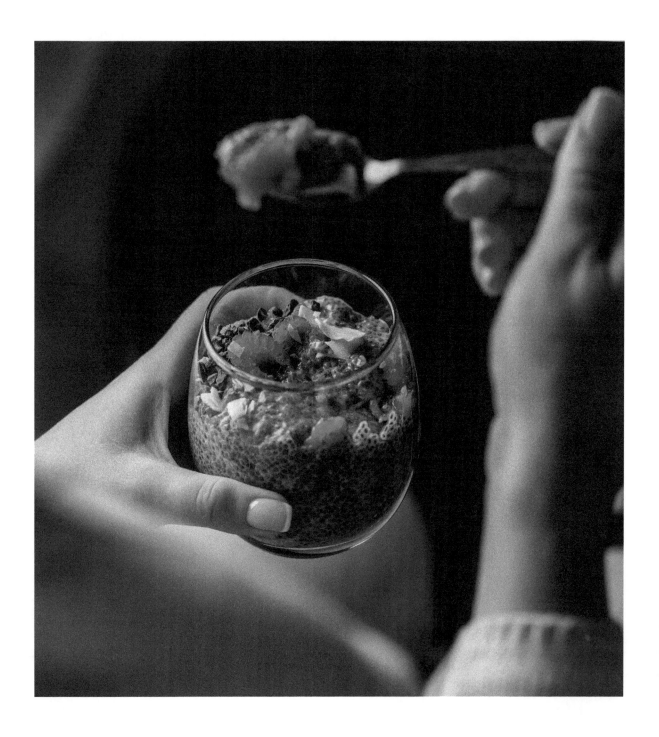

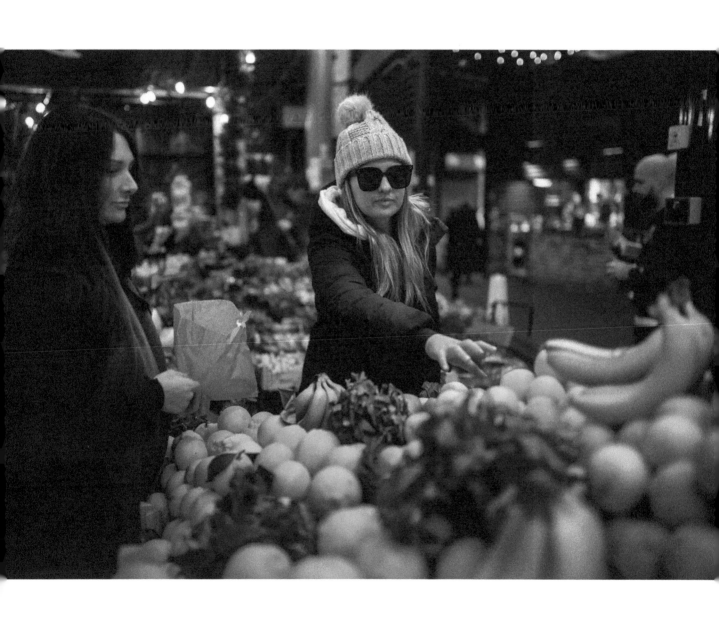

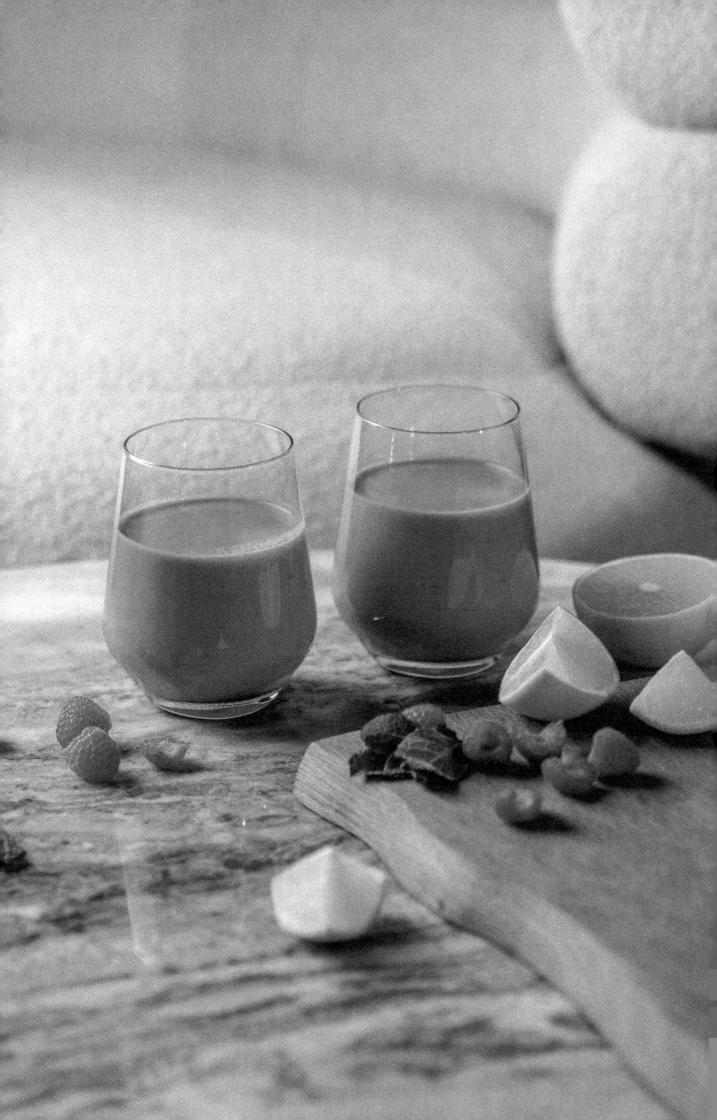

De-stress Raspberry Smoothie

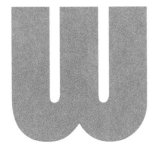ho doesn't need a destress smoothie in their lives? Packed full of antioxidants, protein and fibre. This smoothie is so quick and simple and is just such a lovely, tasty way to stay your day. Zen in a glass!!!

Ingredients
Serves 2

1 cup of frozen raspberries

1 cup of Greek yoghurt or coconut yoghurt

½ cup of any milk of your choice

4 x oranges, juiced

1 banana

2 tbsp honey or maple syrup

Method

1. Put the frozen raspberries, banana, yoghurt and honey/maple syrup in the blender then squeeze in all the juice from the oranges.

2. Blend, look at the consistency, if it needs to be a little looser add some cold water. Enjoy and deeeeeestresss!

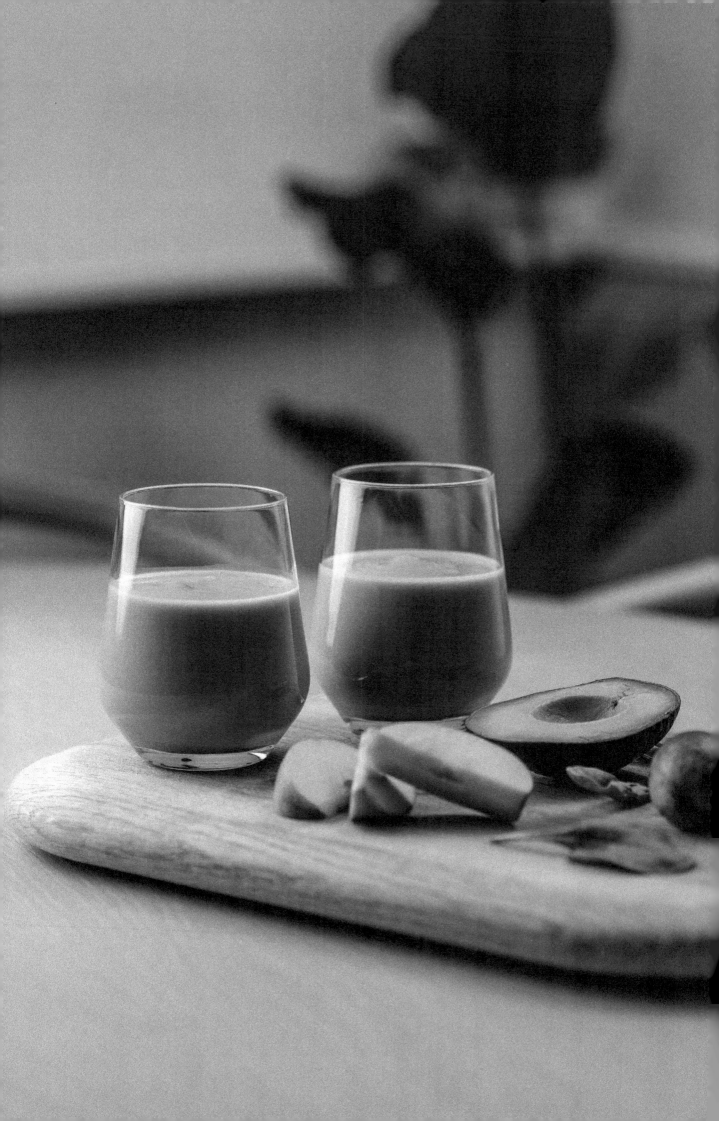

Glow Up Smoothie

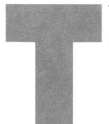This smoothie is the boomb!!!!! Vegan and full of fibre! Get your glow on hunnies!

Ingredients
Serves 2

1 avocado

2 large handful of spinach

100g frozen pineapple

2 green apples

600ml coconut water

Method

1. Peel the apples, core and roughly chop.

2. Then put in the blender along with your avocado, spinach, pineapple and coconut water.

3. Blend until smooth.

This smoothie is sooooo delicious and jam packed full of goodness! xX

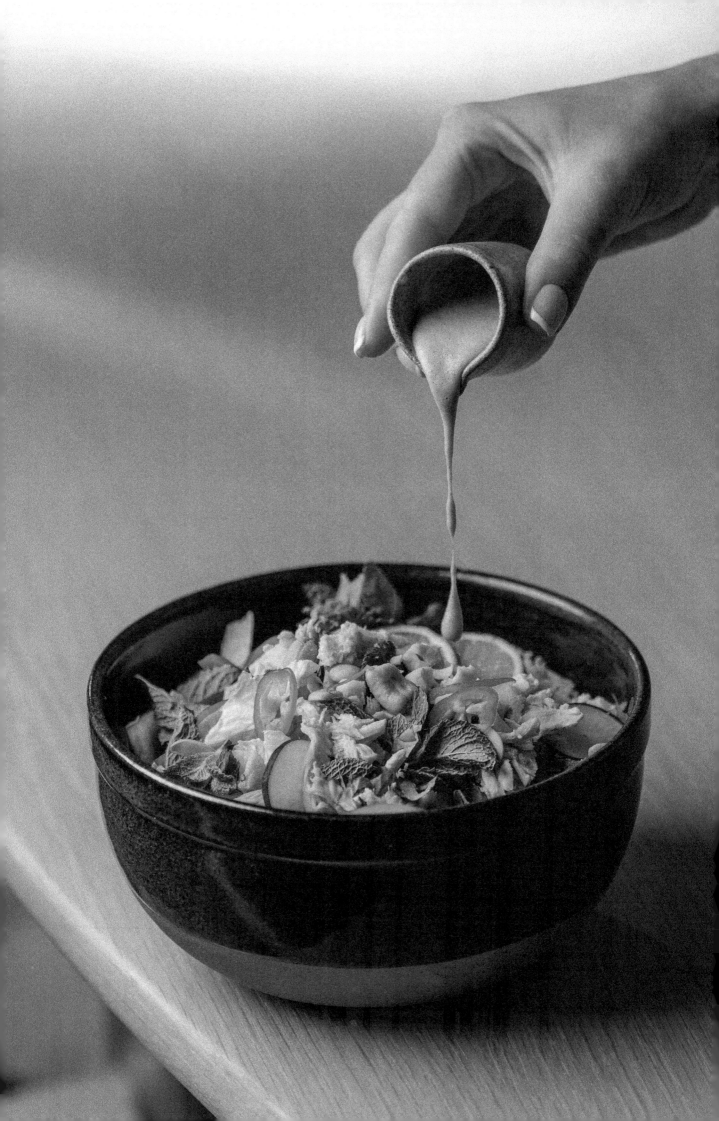

Bang Bang Fridge Raid Salad

This salad is great for using up all the veggies in your fridge! You don't need every single veggie its more inspiration of what you can through in this salad! Its full of colour, flavour and crunchy veggies with a delicious zingy creamy satay dressing! We love this salad so much! P.S. try adding some fresh mango, to bring the tropical vibe for your plate!

Ingredients
Serves 2

Satay salad dressing

2 tbsp peanut butter

2 tbsp soy sauce

Fresh ginger x 1 thumb size piece, peeled and grated

1 tbsp siracha

1 tbsp honey or agave

½ cup of water

2 limes

For the salad

Left over roast chicken (or whichever protein you prefer, tofu, prawns, some leftover cooked beef)

1 carrot, peel and grated

½ cucumber, finely sliced

4 scallions/spring onions, sliced

½ chinese cabbage or gem lettuce, finely shredded (use up

whatever lettuce or spinach you have in your fridge, it will all taste delicious together).

1 red pepper, seeds removed, finely sliced

Handful of radishes, sliced

1 small bunch of fresh cilantro / coriander, roughly chopped

1 small bunch of fresh mint, leaves picked and roughly chopped

1 red chilli finely sliced, optional

1 large handful of roasted nuts, like cashew, peanuts or toasted sesame seeds

1 lime

Method

1. Spoon the peanut butter, soy and chili sauce, ginger, juice of 2 limes, honey or agave and ½ cup of water into your Nutri-Bullet or small blender.

2. Blend all the ingredients until you have a lovely dressing. If it looks a bit thick, add some more water. Set your dressing aside.

3. Add your desired protein to a bowl, if using chicken shred the chicken. Drizzle your protein with some of the yummy satay dressing you have just made. Use just enough to coat your protein so you have lots of dressing left for your salad.

4. Mix the carrot, cucumber, spring onions/scallions, radish, red pepper and lettuce or chines cabbage in a large bowl. Add the coriander and stir through.

5. Add the chicken and dressing to the salad and lightly stir together.

6. Sprinkle the fresh mint leaves, and roasted nuts on top of your salad with chili if using!

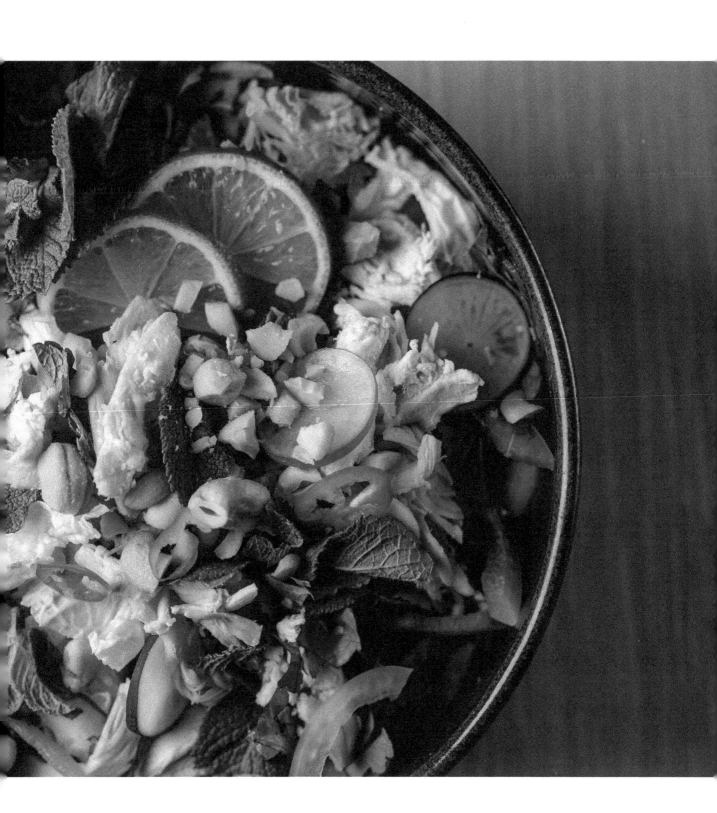

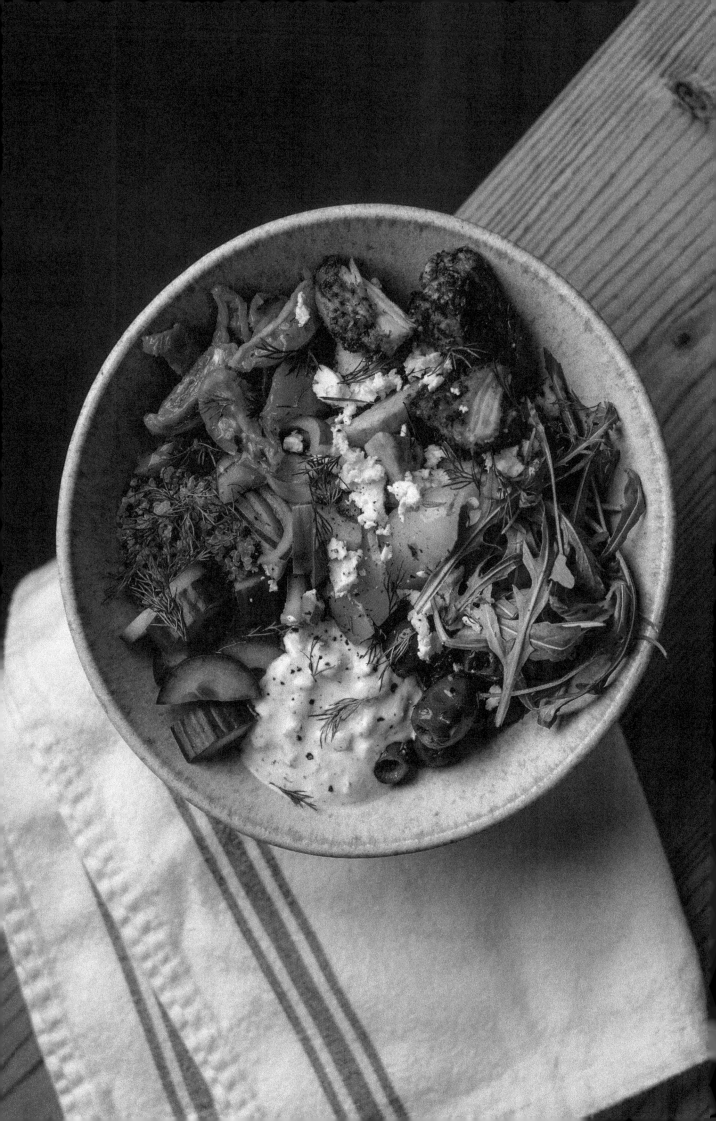

Greek Goddess Bowl

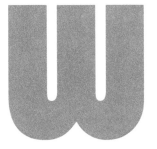e are always on the hunt for lunch dishes that we can pre-prep and don't take hours in the kitchen. You can batch cook your chicken and freeze it or use tofu instead of chicken. We are obsessed with our Greek gyros bowl. It has all the flavours of the traditional Greek classics, filled with marinated chicken, creamy tzatziki, rocket, feta, olives and roasted med vegetables. It keeps SO well and is an amazing lunch to take at work during the week and you can pretend you are on a beautiful Greek island with us!

Ingredients

4 chicken breasts, cut into dice

1 lemon

1 tsp of oregano, paprika, cumin

Fresh thyme, rosemary, dill and mint

1tub of tzatziki

Feta

Olives

1 jar of mixed roasted peppers (I use red and yellow)

2 red onions

1 packet of rocket

1 packet of cooked quinoa

4 tomatoes or a packet of cherry tomatoes or sundried tomatoes

1 cucumber

Olive oil

Salt and pepper

Method

1. Preheat your oven to 335F/170C.

2. Mix the juice of one lemon, 1 tbsp olive oil, 1 tbsp oregano, 1 tbsp paprika, 2 tsp cumin, 2 tsp salt, black pepper, fresh thyme and rosemary, 2 cloves of minced garlic.

3. Coat your chicken or tofu with the marinade and put on a lined baking tray and cook in the oven for 20-25 minutes until the chicken is cooked through but lovely and juicy.

4. Roughly chop your cucumber, tomatoes, peppers and red onions. Toss in a little olive oil, salt, pepper and a squeeze of lemon juice.

5. Start to assemble your bowl. Base of quinoa, rocket, olives, tomatoes, cucumber, peppers, crumbled feta, chicken or tofu and a good dollop of tzatziki. Roughly chop your mint and dill to sprinkle on top of your bowl and enjoy this nourishing bowl which will hopefully transport you to a Greek island in the sunshine.

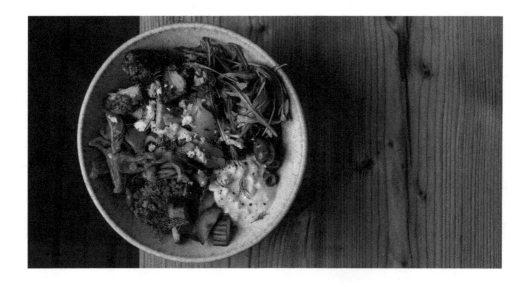

Bryony Johnson & Daisy Kellihe

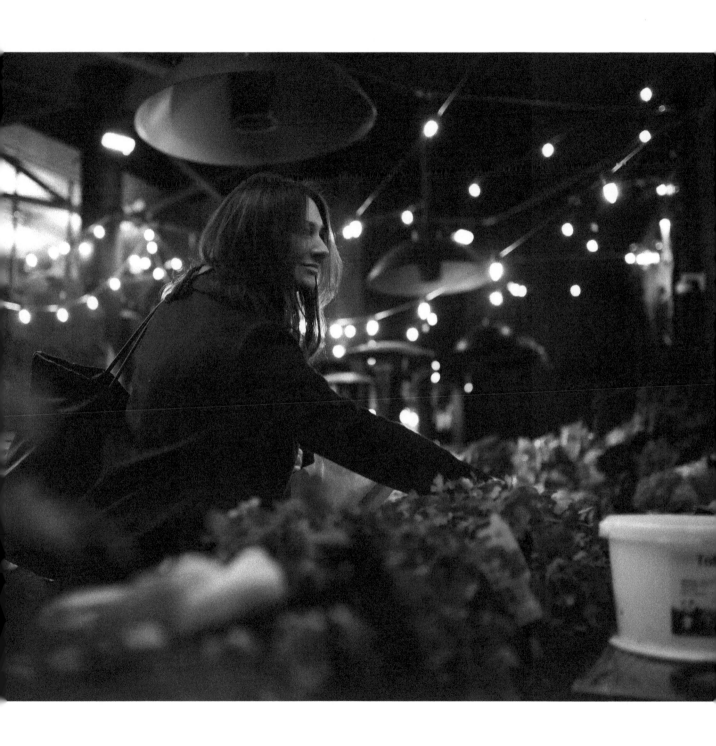

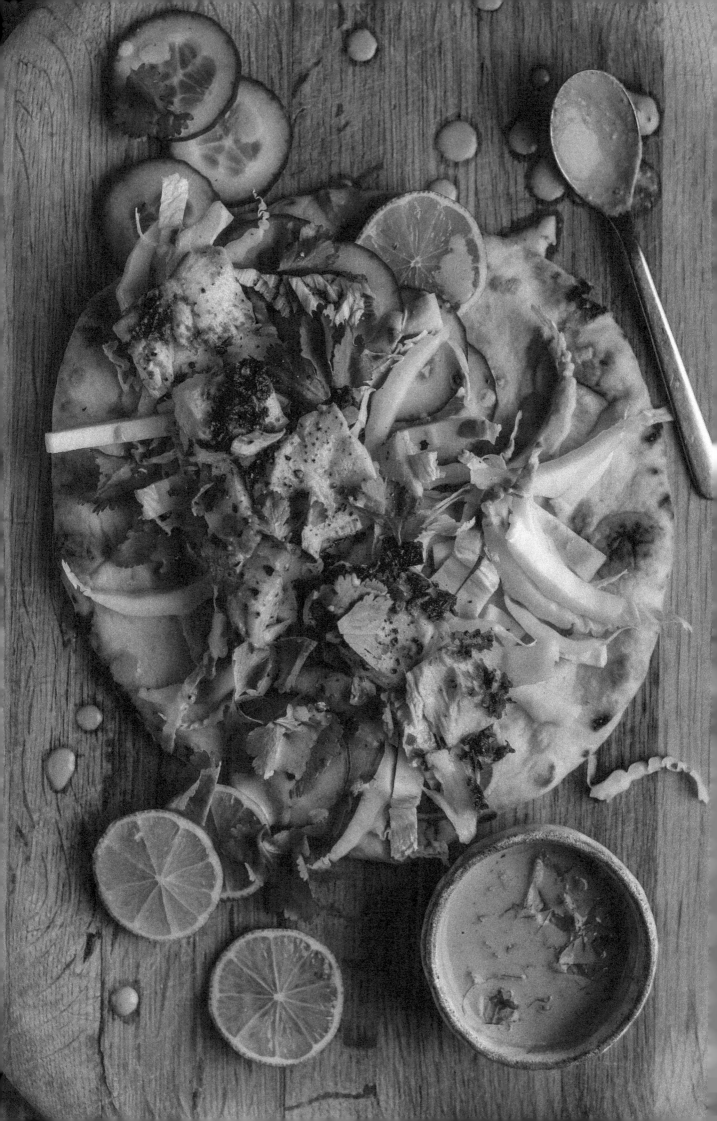

Harissa Salmon Flat Breads

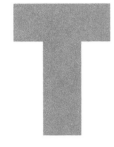

These are always a yacht crew's favourite, they are like a healthy burrito! Full of freshness and flavour! You could always substitute the salmon for halloumi or tofu, and they would be damn delicious! Simple and speedy to make, this will become one of your weekly favourites

Ingredients
Serves 2

2 multi seeded flat breads

2 salmon fillets

2 tbsp harissa

¼ cucumber, sliced

¼ white cabbage, shredded or baby spinach or rocket

½ red onion, thinly sliced

Handful of fresh coriander

Handful of fresh mint leaves

Olive oil

Salt and pepper

Herby tahini dressing

2 tbsp tahini

2 tbsp plain yogurt or plant-based alternative

1 tbsp jalapenos more for extra spice

Juice of 1 lemon

Large handful of fresh mint leaves

Two large handfuls of fresh coriander

Salt and pepper

Method

1. Pre heat the oven to 350F / 180C. Line a baking tray with baking paper. Put the salmon fillets on the tray drizzle with a little oil, season with salt and pepper, then brush each salmon fillet with 1tbsp of harissa paste.

2. Cook the fillets in the oven for 15 minutes.

3. Sprinkle the flatbreads with a little water and grill for 2 minutes.

4. Shred your white cabbage and thinly slice your cucumber and red onion. Roughly chop the fresh coriander and mint.

5. Take your small blender, put all the tahini dressing ingredients into the blender and blend until smooth. If it needs a little water to loosen it up add a little cold water.

6. To assemble the flat breads, fill them with the shredded cabbage or spinach, then flake the salmon, sliced cucumber, red onion, fresh herbs and a drizzle of the tahini herby dressing or left over tzatziki and sit down and enjoy!

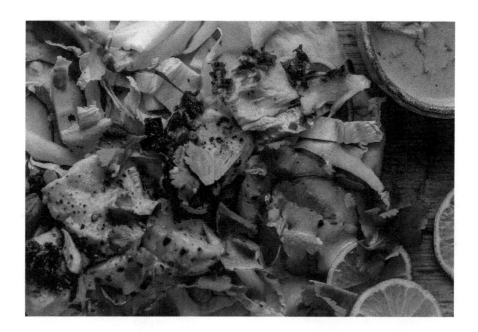

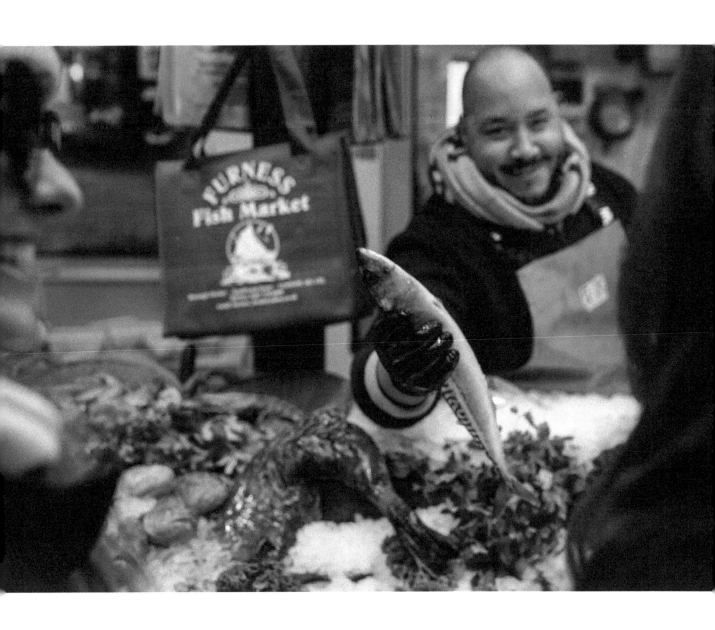

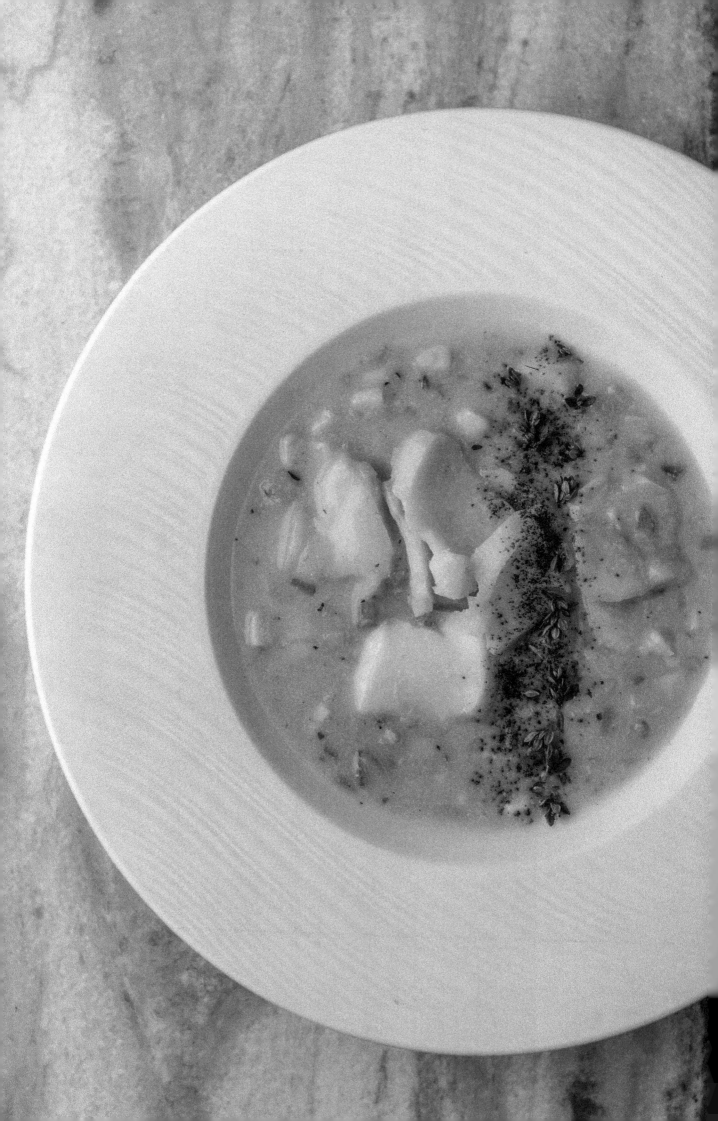

Healthy Hearty Smoked Haddock Chowder

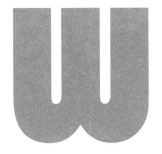 e could eat this soup all year round! Full of veggies and beautiful smoked fish, it always hits the spot! Quite simply a super nourishing bowl of goodness! And its so addictive!

Ingredients
Serves 2 (with a little left over)

200g/8oz smoked cod or haddock (undyed)

1 tbsp olive oil

1 small onion, finely chopped

2 leeks, finely chopped

2 celery sticks, thinly sliced

60g / 2oz tinned or frozen corn

200g / 8oz potato, peeled and diced

2 cloves of garlic, finely chopped

1 tsp chopped fresh thyme or 1tsp dried thyme

500ml / 17.5oz of milk

Fresh parsley or chives, chopped

Pinch cayenne pepper optional

Zest of 1 lemon

Salt and pepper

Method

1. Put the fish in a deep frying pan with 700ml of boiling water. Cover and simmer for 2 minutes. Turn off the heat and leave to stand, covered, for a further 5 minutes. Drain, reserving the liquid, then flake the fish.

2. Heat the oil in a deep saucepan. Add the vegetables and garlic and sauté over a medium heat until the veggies start to soften. Stir in the thyme and the reserved cooking liquid and bring to the boil. Reduce the heat and simmer for 10 minutes until the vegetables have softened. The potatoes must be cooked through.

3. Pour half the soup into a bowl and mash with a potato masher or fork. Return to the pan with the milk, fish and lemon zest. Simmer for 3 minutes, until everything is hot to trot! taste and season if needed. Sprinkle with chopped parsley or chives and a sprinkle of cayenne pepper (if using).

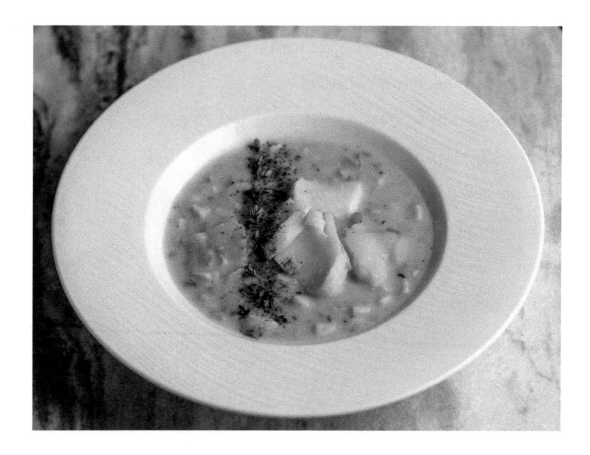

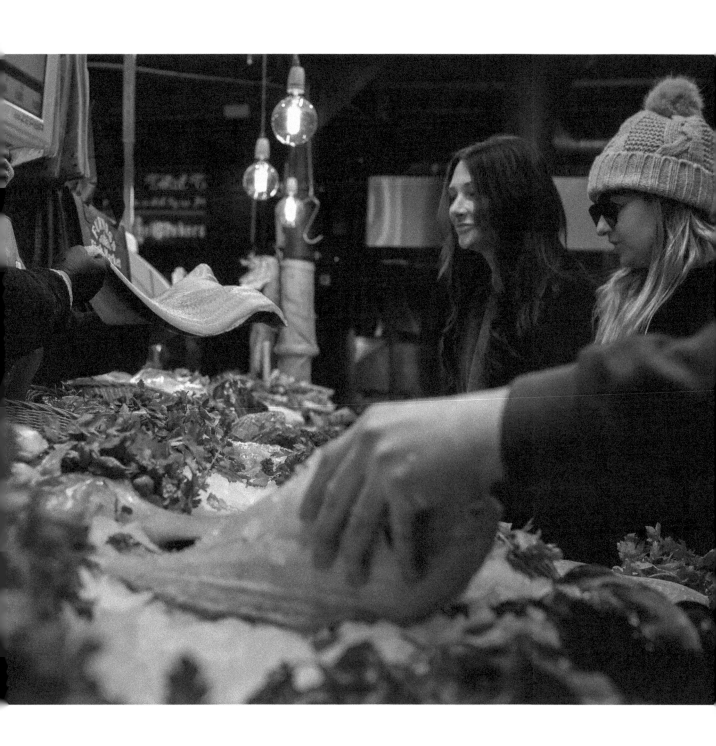

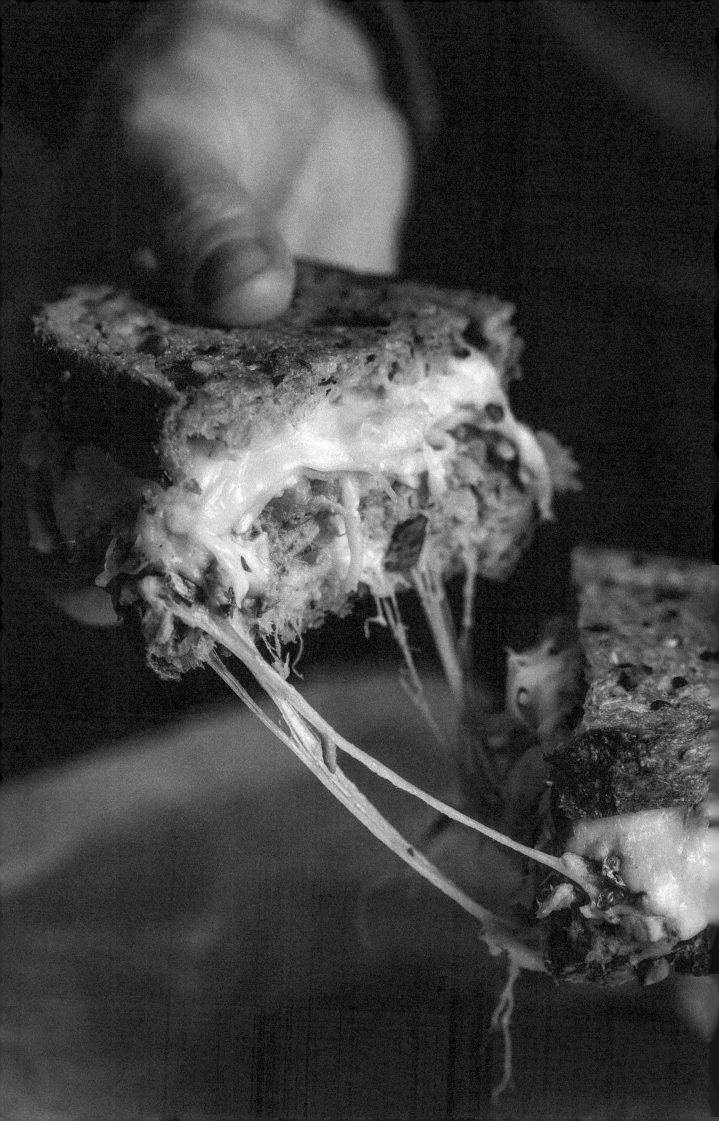

Healthy Tuna Melt

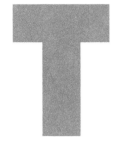

There is something about a tuna melt that just... hits the spot! It is one of my favourite sandwiches and this is our healthier version with a lighter tuna no mayo mix and pesto toast. Be warned, this could be your new lunch obsession.

Ingredients

Serves 2

2 tins of tuna in brine or water

2 heaped tbsp Greek yoghurt

2 tbsp pesto

Zest of 1 lemon

Pinch of salt and pepper

2 tbsp of jalapeños (if you like a little spice)

4 slices of bread of choice, we used seeded sourdough

2 tomatoes, sliced

1/4 red onion, sliced (optional)

2 tsp extra virgin olive oil

Fresh parsley or basil

80g / 3oz of cheese of choice, we used mozzarella, but you could use, cheddar, gruyere or any cheese of your fancy!

Method

1. Drain the tuna well. Mix the tuna with yoghurt, pesto, lemon zest, jalapenos (if using), herbs and season with salt and pepper.

2. Brush one side of your bread lightly with your olive oil, flip the

bread over and start to fill the bread with the tuna mix. Slice the tomatoes and lay over the tuna along with the sliced red onions, sliced cheese, and press the sandwich together.

3. If you have an air fryer, cook at 200c for 3 minutes on each side until golden brown or in a frying pan, cook on a medium heat on either side for 4 minutes.

4. Cut in half and dive in, pure heaven!

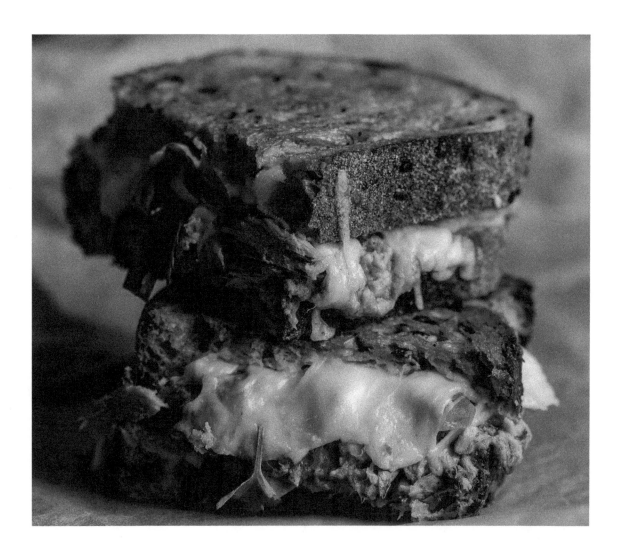

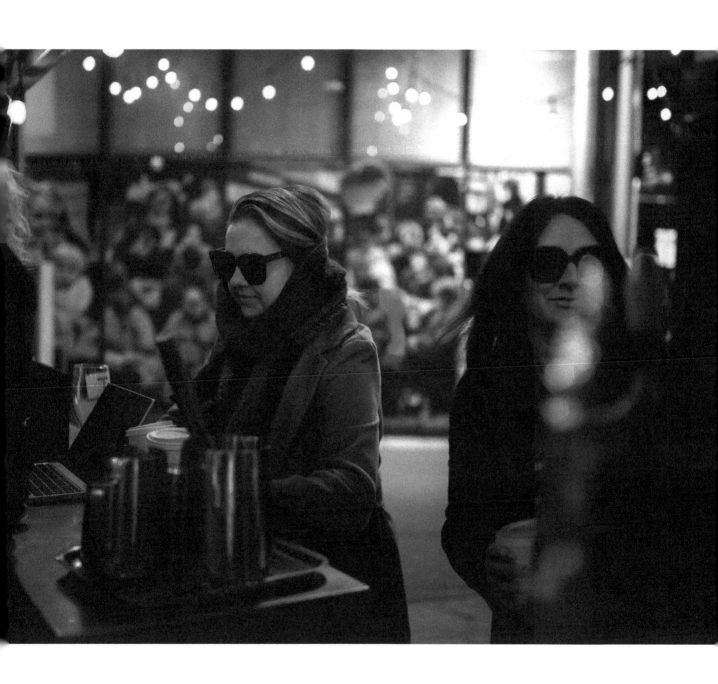

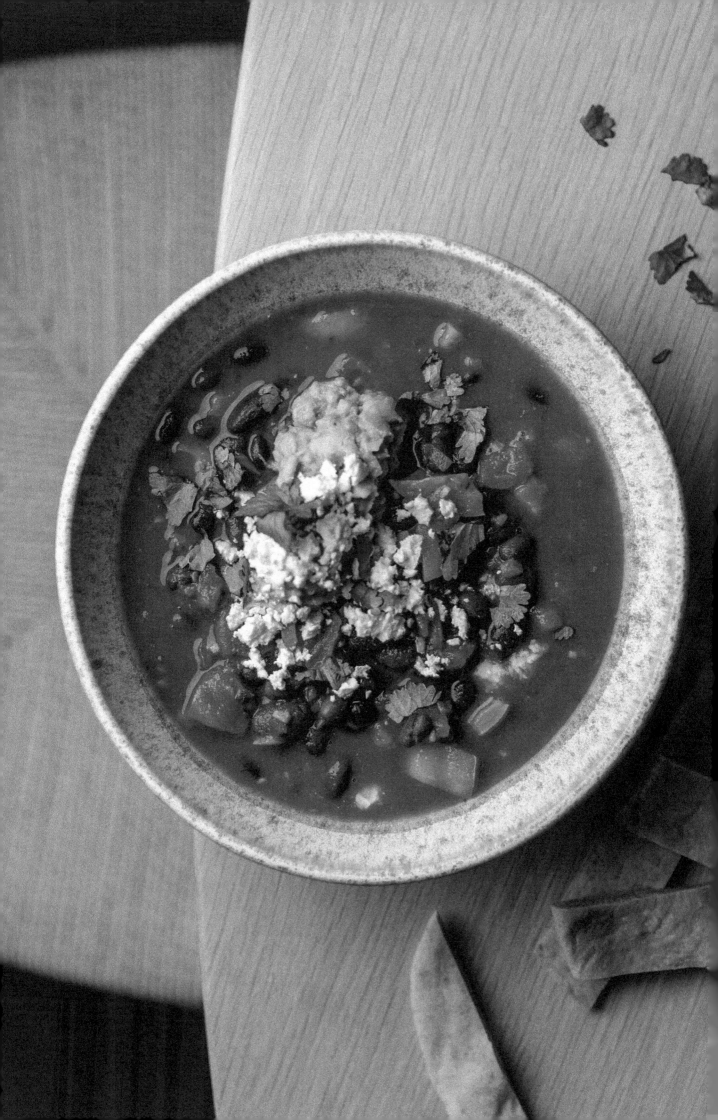

Mexican Bean Soup

This soup is packed full of flavour and protein. It is so healthy and makes us feel that even when we are crossing the Atlantic, it brings the flavours of Mexico into the galley! This soup freezes so well, and great to batch cook and freeze portions, so you have a ready made meal for when you get home and don't have time to cook.

Ingredients
Serves 4

1 tbsp olive oil

1 large onion, chopped

1 red pepper, cut into chunks

1 yellow pepper, cut into chucks

2 cloves of garlic

2 tsp chipotle paste or seasoning or chili powder

2 tsp ground coriander

2 tsp ground cumin

1 tin of chopped tomatoes

1 can/400g black beans

1 can/400g kidney beans

1 vegetable or vegan stock cube

1 small avocado

Large handful of fresh coriander, roughly chopped

1 lime, juiced

2 tbsp jalapenos, chopped

Feta or plant-based alternative

Method

1. Heat the oil in a medium pan, on a medium to low heat, add the onion (reserving 1 tbsp to make the guacamole later) and pepper and fry, stirring frequently, for 10 mins. Stir in the garlic and spices, then tip in the tomatoes and beans with their liquid, half a can of water and the stock cube. Simmer, covered, for 20 mins.

2. Meanwhile, peel and de-stone the avocado and tip into a bowl, add the remaining onion, coriander and lime juice with your chopped jalapeños (if using) and mash well. Ladle the soup into your bowls, top with the guacamole and sprinkle with some feta and you have got a bowl full of protein and flavour! Sit down and enjoy!

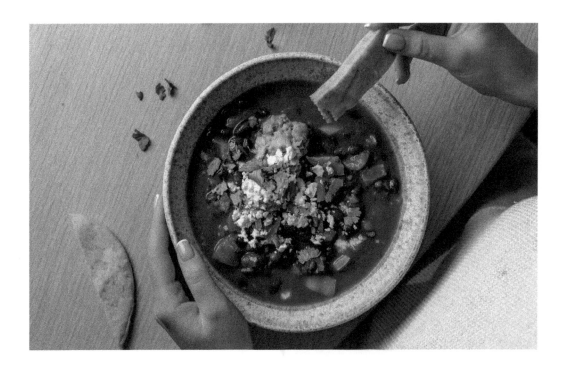

Bryony Johnson & Daisy Kellihe

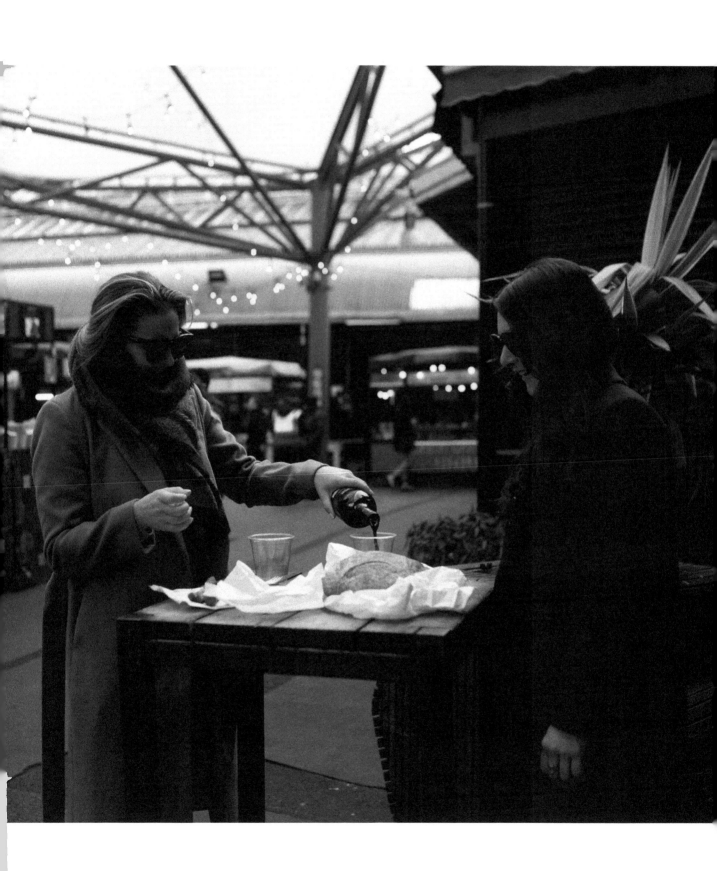

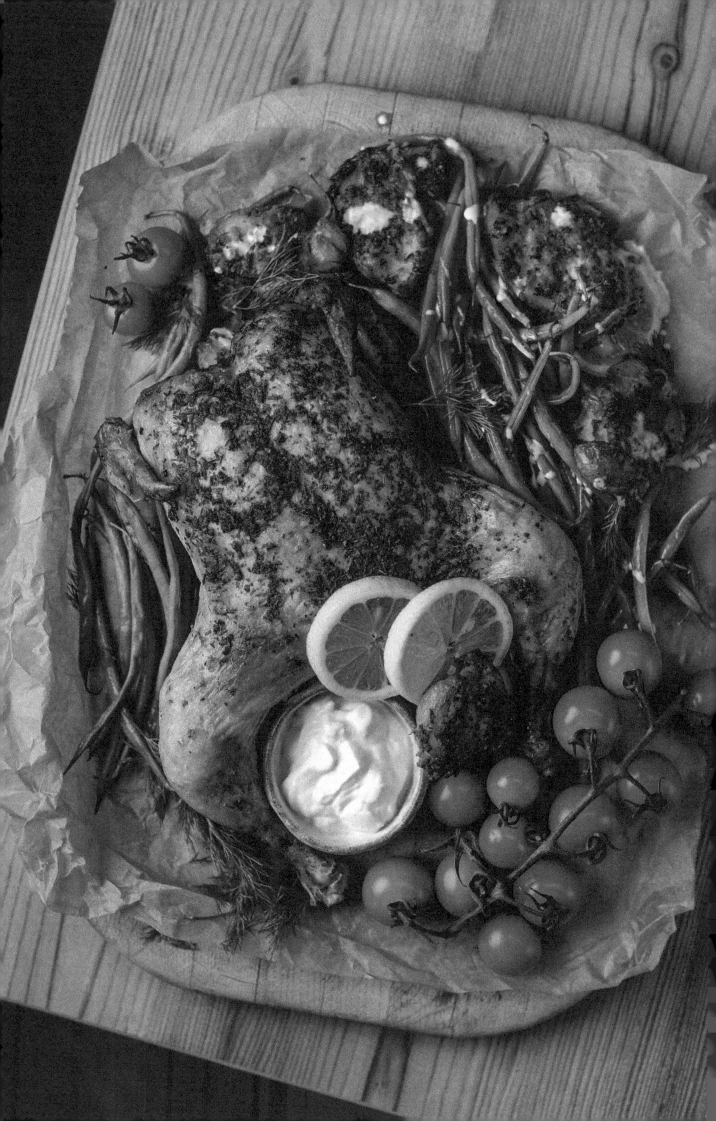

Roasted Chicken, Smashed Parmesan Potatoes with Green Beans, Harissa, Yoghurt and Dill

his is such a great relaxed meal to invite friends around for! Put everything in the middle of the table and let everyone help themselves. Get the wine flowing and enjoy good food and friends.

Ingredients
Serves 4

1 whole chicken

700g / 24oz new potatoes

2 lemons, zested

1 tbsp thyme

3 tbsp olive oil

2 tbsp fresh rosemary, finely chopped

1 tbsp oregano

4 cloves of garlic

50g parmesan

300g / 10oz green beans

3 tbsp harissa

3 tbsp yogurt

Small bunch of fresh dill optional

Salt and pepper

Method

1. Heat oven to 335F / 170C fan. Have a shelf ready in the middle of the oven without any shelves above it.

2. Take your chicken out of the fridge 30 mins before you want to cook it so it can come up to room temperature. Pat the chicken dry with some kitchen paper. Drizzle the chicken with 1tbsp olive oil and rub the oil all over the chicken, season with salt and pepper. Rub the thyme and oregano into the chicken.

3. Chop 1 of the lemons into quarters and put into the chicken's cavity with 3 cloves of garlic, bashed a little so that lovely garlicy flavour with come out. Roast in the oven for 1 ½ hours, undisturbed. This should give you a perfectly roasted chicken. To check, pierce the thigh with a skewer and the juices should run clear.

4. While the chicken is cooking get your new potatoes put into a pan of cold salted water, bring to the boil and cook for 15-20 minutes until tender and falling off the end of a knife when poked. While they are cooking mix the parmesan, rosemary, 1 clove of garlic grated, 2 tbsp olive oil, salt and pepper in a large bowl. Drain the potatoes and place them in the bowl with the parmesan and coat all the potatoes in the mixture. Tip the potatoes onto a large baking tray, then using the base of a mug or anything similar, gently squash the spud down so it burst open and place in the oven with the chicken for 20-25 minutes.

5. When the chicken is ready let it rest for 10 minutes, while the chicken is resting cook the green beans in boiling salted water for 4-5 mins until tender. Drain the beans then drizzle with a little olive oil the lemon zest, salt and pepper.

6. Serve your chicken up with your delicious parmesan potatoes, zesty green beans dolloped with some harissa, yogurt and a

sprinkling of chopped dill (or any herbs you like). Dig into this healthy yummy alternative roast!

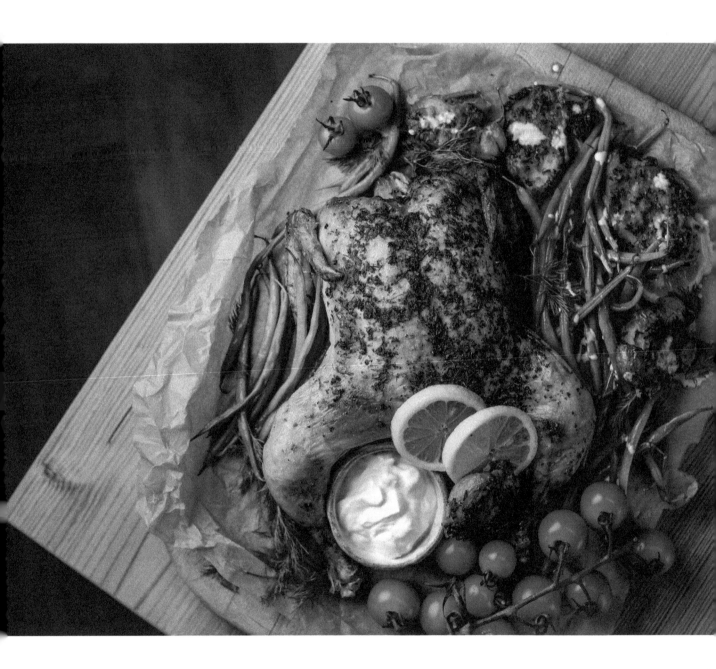

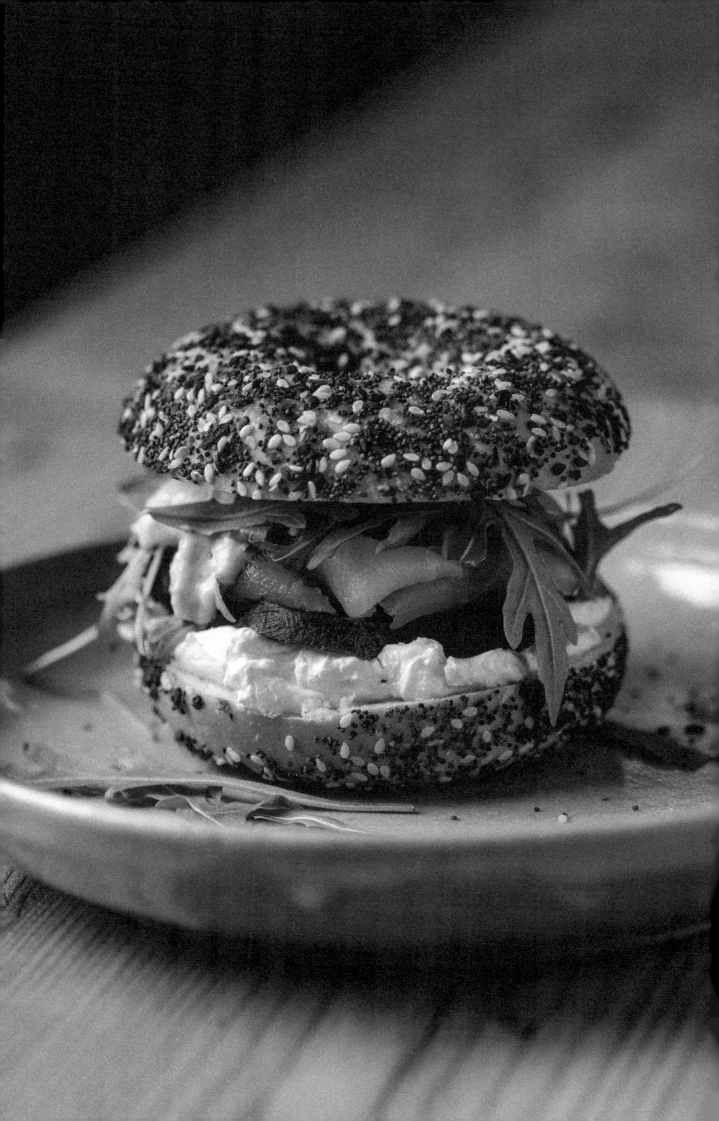

Smoked Salmon and Cream Cheese Bagel

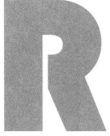**R**eady in minutes, you can eat this for breakfast, brunch or lunch! Super simple but oh so tasty. Little tip is to wear some gloves when slicing your beetroot, so you don't look like you have just committed a crime in the kitchen!

Ingredients
Serves 2

2 multi seeded bagel thins

4 slices of smoked salmon

2 cooked beetroot

2 tsp creamed horseradish

2 tbsp ½ fat cream cheese

2 handfuls of rocket

1/2 lemon

pepper

Method

1. Toast your bagels. While your bagels are toasting slice your beetroot.

2. Get you toasted bagels and spread with horseradish, cream cheese, your sliced beetroot, two slices of smoked salmon a little squeeze of lemon and some freshly ground pepper, a handful of rocket on top!

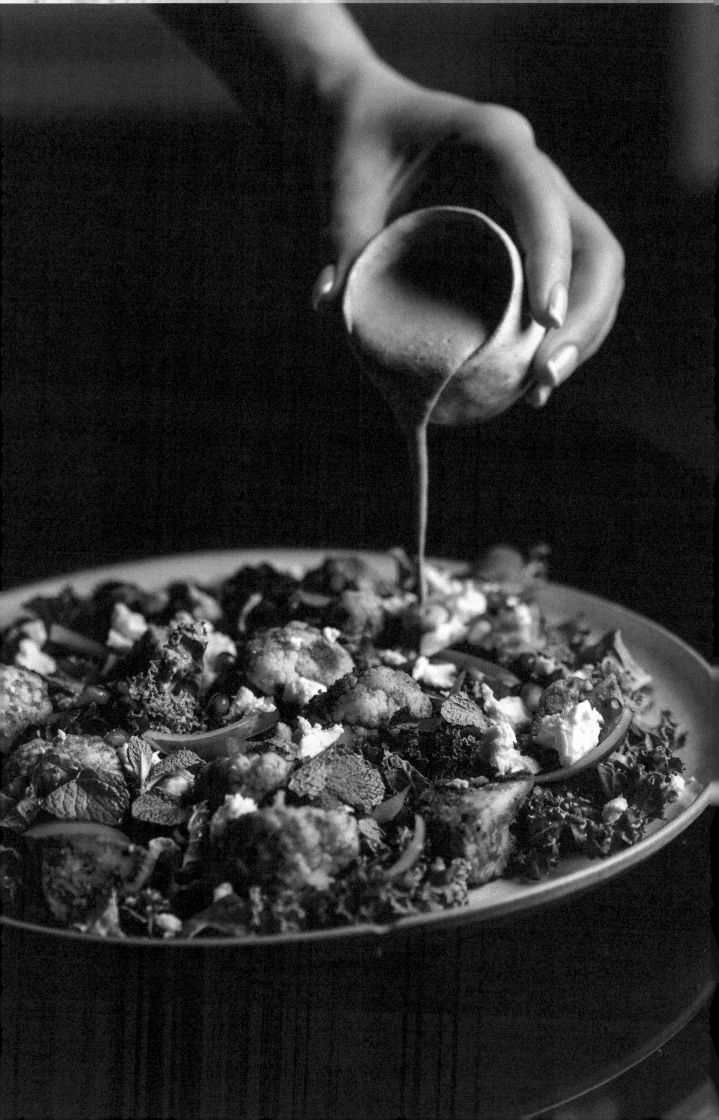

Tandoori Cauliflower Salad

This is one sexy salad, so many textures and flavour, and there are some serious chef kisses with the herby tahini dressing. You can use the dressing over everything! We like to use it for a healthier chicken cesar salad. If you want to add your favourite protein to this salad, go for it!

Ingredients
Serves 2

½ cauliflower

1 bag or bunch of kale

½ a red onion, sliced

½ cup of pomegranate seeds

1 can of cooked chickpeas, drained

Feta or plant based alternative

½ jar of pickled red cabbage, drained

Fresh mint or coriander or both, roughly chopped

1 tbsp curry powder

Olive oil

Herby tahini dressing

2 tbsp tahini

2 tbsp plain yoghurt or plant based alternative

1 tbsp jalapenos more for extra spice

Juice of 1 lemon

Large handful of fresh mint leaves

Two large handfuls of fresh coriander

Salt and pepper

Method

1. Pre heat the oven to 335F / 170C. Line a baking tray with baking parchment paper.

2. Cut up the cauliflower into florets, put onto your baking tray, drizzle your cauliflower with a little olive oil and sprinkle the curry powder over the cauliflower and mix all the oil and curry powder into the cauliflower with your hands. Then season with salt and pepper, place into the oven for 15-20 minutes.

3. Remove the large stalks from your kale, then shred the kale and in a large mixing bowl, place the kale in the bowl, sprinkle with a good pinch of salt and a little drizzle of olive oil. Now really scrunch (massage) the kale with your hands as this breaks down the kale so when you eat it's not chewy but delicious.

4. Take your nutribullet or small blender, put all the tahini dressing ingredients into the blender and blend until smooth. If it needs a little water to loosen it up add a little cold water. Set aside.

5. Right let's start putting the salad together! Start with your kale, then are your roasted cauliflower, pickled red onion, sliced red onion, pomegranate seeds, crumble your feta, then scatter with your herbs and drizzle that gorgeous herby tahini dressing on top! Wow just Wow!

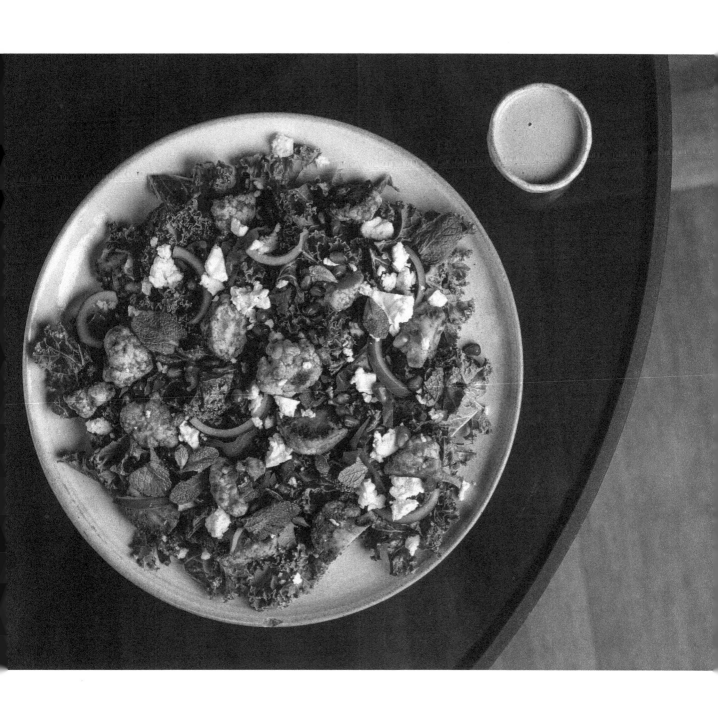

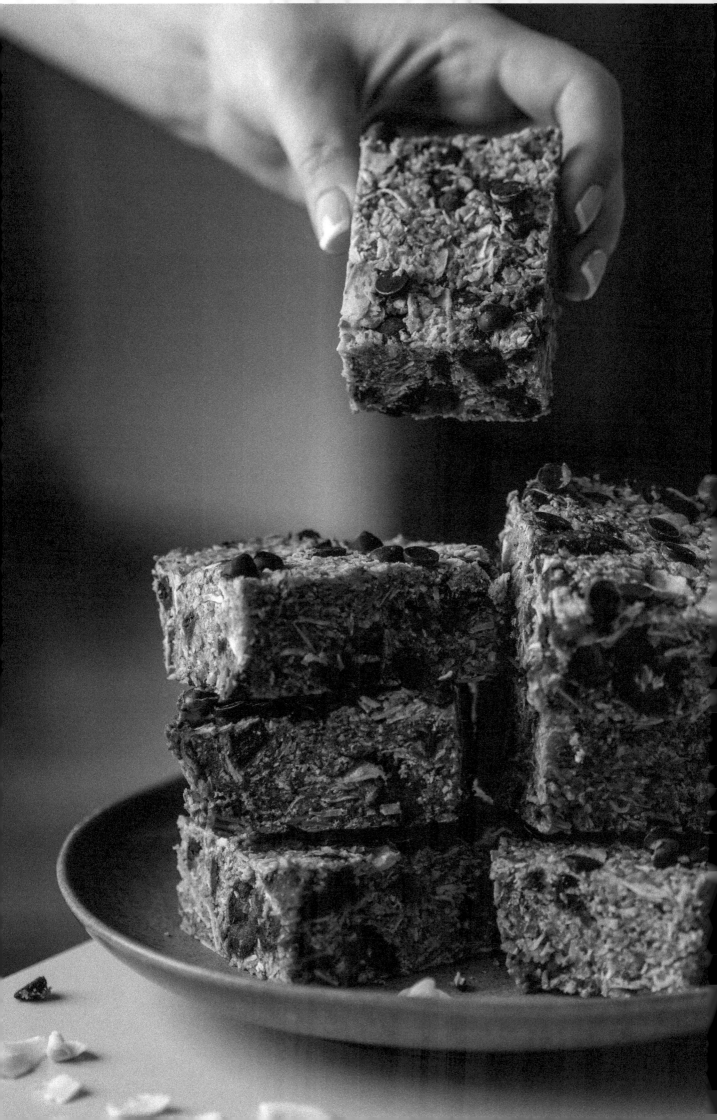

Banana, Coconut Oat Bars

These bars will quickly become a firm favourite in your home! So simple to make and good to batch cook. They are great to have as a snack pre or post work out, or any time of the day for that matter, we sometimes have them on the go for breakfast! They have lots of slow release energy, are packed full of goodness and damn delicious! Enjoy these bars as they are mighty fine!

Ingredients
Makes 10 Bars

9.7oz/275g oats

2 tbsp ground flax seed

½ tsp salt

1/2cup / 30g unsweetened coconut flakes

1tsp cinnamon

1 tsp vanilla

1 cup / 240ml milk or plant-based milk of your choice

3 ripe bananas, mashed

5 medjool dates, finely chopped

2 tbsp maple syrup

1/2 cup dark chocolate chips, or vegan chocolate for topping, optional

Method

1. Pre-heat oven to 340F/170 C

2. Add the oats, flax, coconut, salt and cinnamon to a bowl and stir

to combine.

3. Mash the banana in a bowl using a fork until it forms a thick, chunky paste.

4. Add the milk, vanilla, banana, dates and vegan choc chips if using to the oat mixture and stir into a thick batter.

5. Taste the batter and if you feel like you want it a little sweeter, add 1-2 tbsp maple syrup.

6. Line an approximately 7–8-inch square baking pan with parchment paper, add the oat mixture to the pan and flatten out until even.

7. Bake for 20-25 minutes.

8. Leave to cool before slicing into squares or large bars.

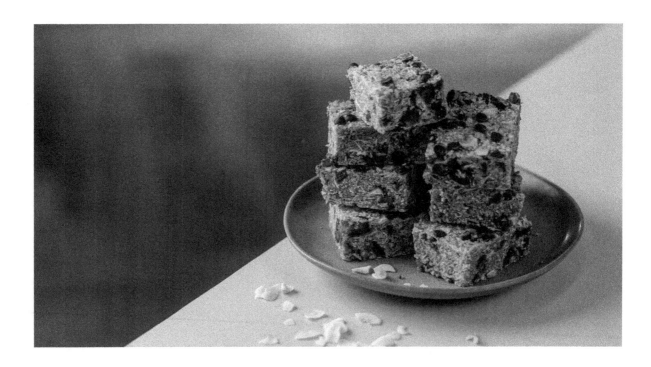

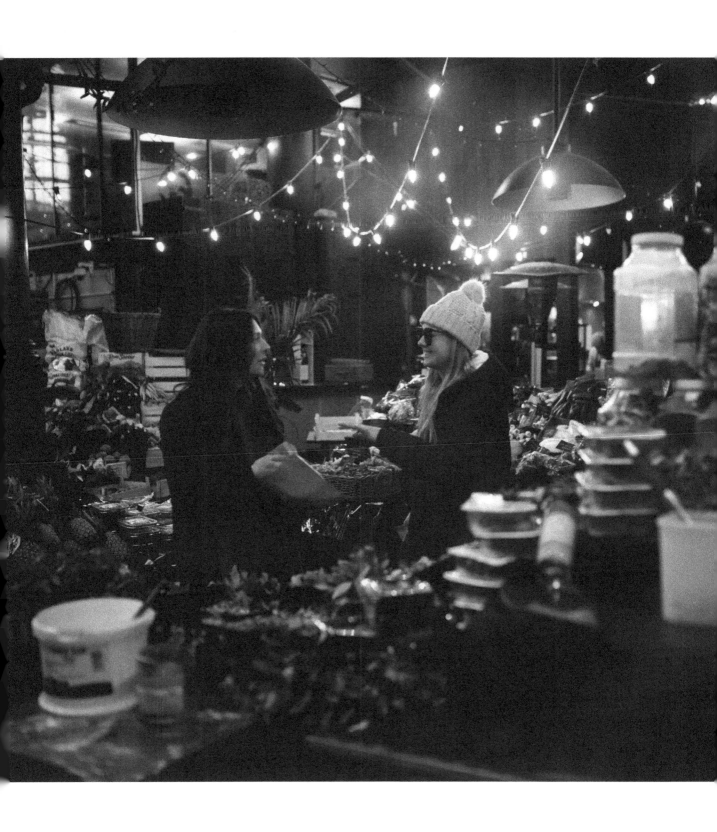

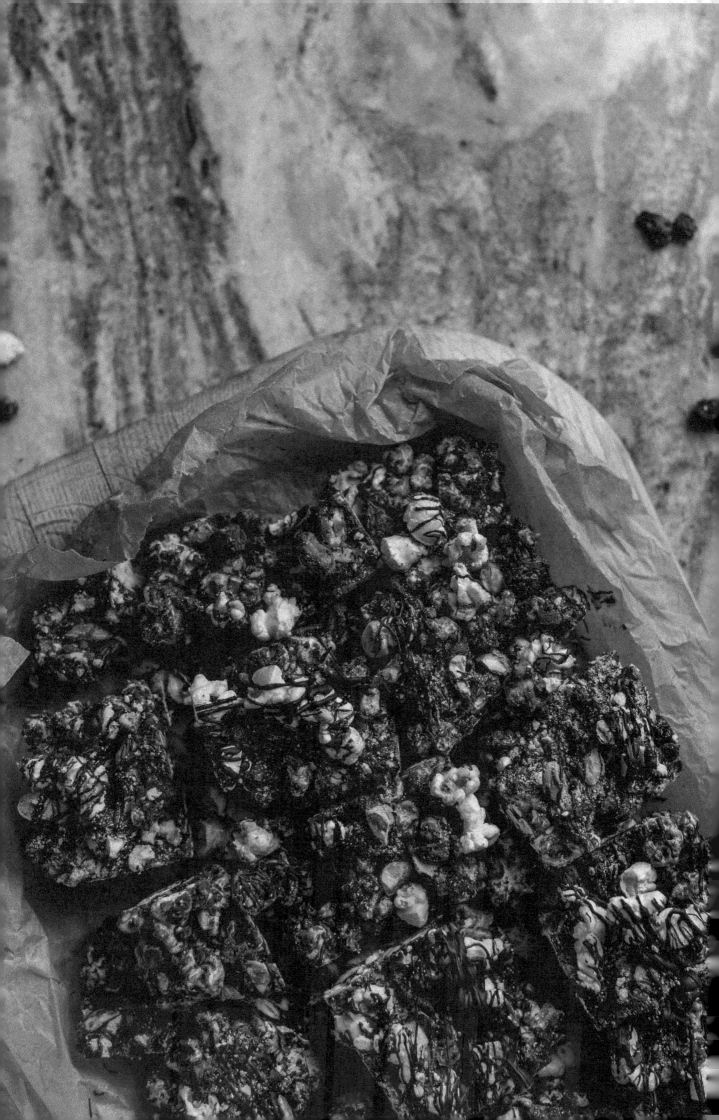

Healthy Rocky Roads

That's right, healthy rocky road bars! If we could give you two pieces of advice, the first would be wear sunscreen and the second would be, make these bars and put them straight into the freezer or you will eat them all in one go! But hopefully you have more will power than us!

Ingredients
Makes 12 squares

200g / 7oz Dark chocolate

1 cup of nut butter

2 tbsp coconut oil

2 tbsp maple Syrup

½ cup roasted pistachios

½ roasted almonds

1/3 cup dried cranberries

2 cups of plain popcorn

Method

1. Line a square brownie tin with baking paper, slightly grease the tin then line with the baking paper and set aside.

2. In a saucepan, under a low heat, melt the dark chocolate, nut butter, coconut oil, maple syrup. When the chocolate has melted remove from the heat.

3. Stir in the nuts, popcorn, dried cranberries. Make sure all the ingredients are mixed together and transfer to the prepared tin. Press the mixture down with the back of a silicon spatula so that the mixture is spread and flattened evenly.

4. Set in the fridge for 1 hour to set. Cut into 12 squares. These squares are great to keep in the freezer and can be eaten straight from the freezer!

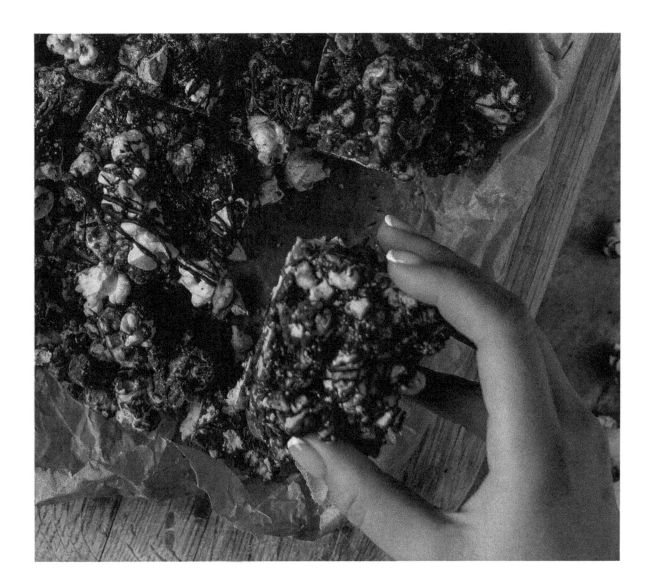

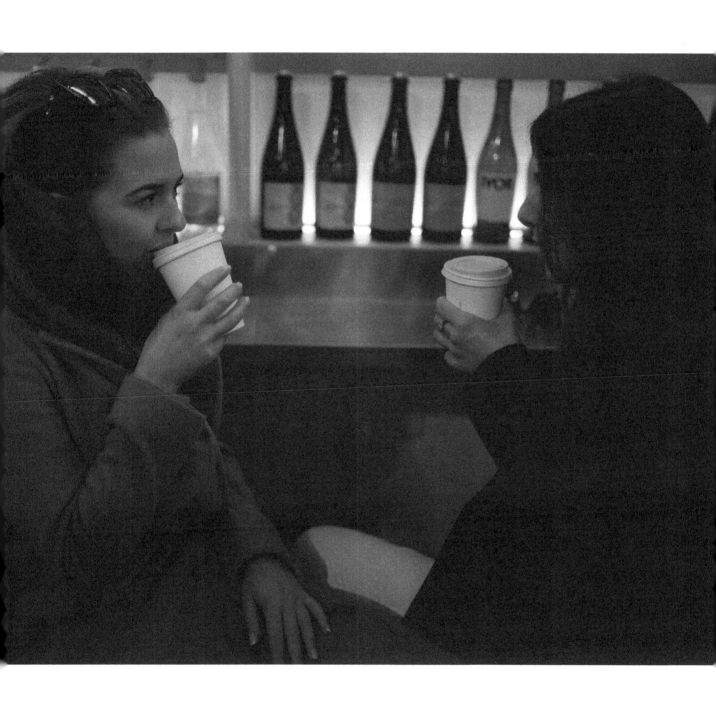

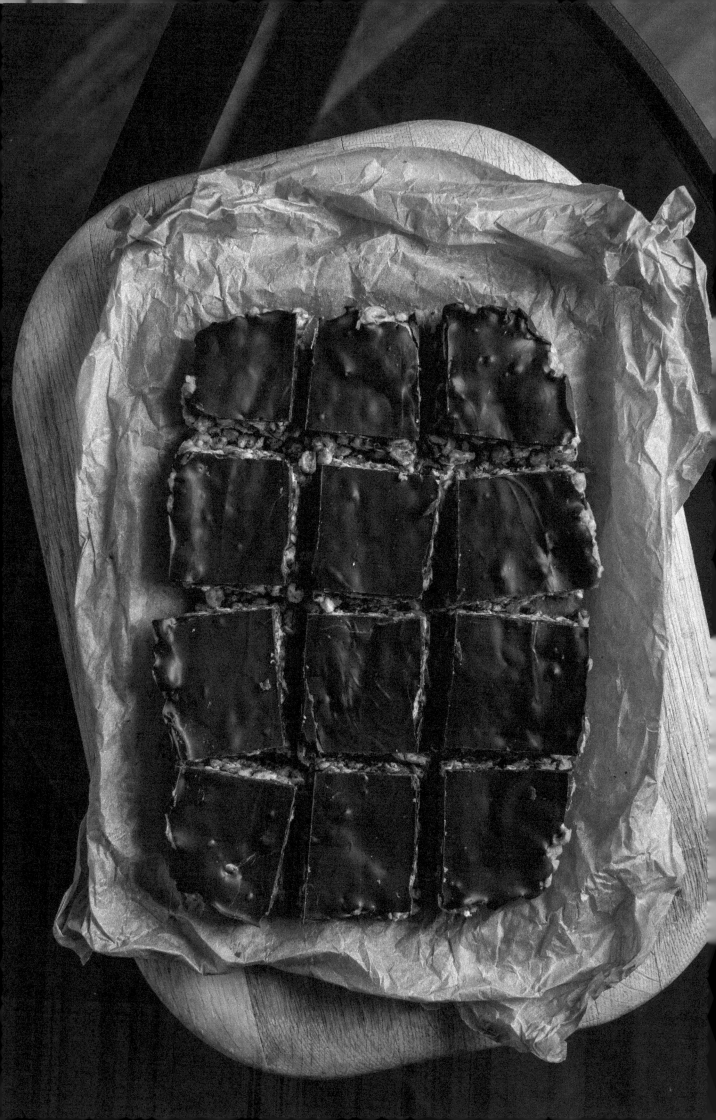

The OG Rice Crispy Bars

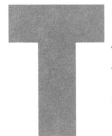his is a nutritious galley girls twist on an OG classic! Addictive does not even come close. Put a lock on that fridge or just go with our rule... if it's not on a plate the calories don't count. Simple!

Ingredients
Makes 12

100g / 4oz of rice cakes, crushed

4 tbsp maple syrup

200g / 7oz peanut butter

Big pinch of salt

200g / 7oz dark chocolate

Method

1. In a bowl crush the rice cakes, break down into small pieces.

2. In a small pan melt your maple syrup, peanut butter and a pinch of salt. Then pour into your crushed rice cakes and mix well.

3. Grease a brownie tin then line with parchment paper.

4. Empty the rice mixture into the lined baking tin and flatten down evenly.

5. Melt the dark chocolate on a low heat in a non-stick frying pan. Pour the melted chocolate over the rice mixture covering the whole surface.

6. Place the tin in the fridge for 1 hour to set. Then slice into 12 squares. These are great to keep in the fridge or freezer! Yum bums!

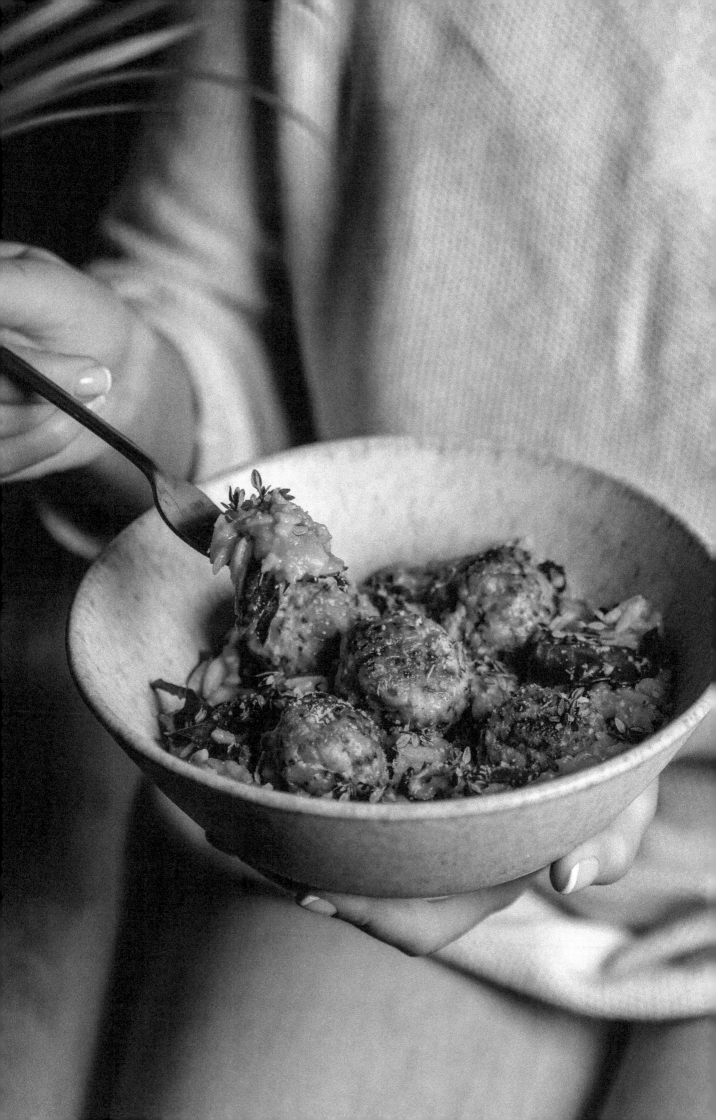

Baked Rosemary Chicken Meatballs with Tomato Orzo

This dish is so great and easy to cook, satisfying and damn delicious. A great thing to do is to batch cook the chicken meatballs. You can also use the chicken meatballs in a Greek goodness bowl on page () for your lunch the next day! You could also try using mince turkey instead of chicken, to mix things up. They freeze well, so you have something quick and healthy in the freezer for those weeks were time flies by. I batch cook a whole load of meatballs for an Atlantic crossing and are always a favourite with a hungry crew who are the toughest crowd! x

Ingredients
Serves 4

Meatballs

1 1/2 lbs/500g minced chicken

2 oz/50g breadcrumbs

1 tsp granulated garlic

1 tsp chilli flakes (optional)

1 cup sundried tomatoes, in oil chopped

2 tbsp fresh Italian parsley chopped

2 tbsp fresh rosemary finely chopped

1 tbsp olive oil

Salt and pepper

Tomato orzo

1 tbsp olive oil

2 shallots, finely chopped

4 cloves garlic, minced

2 cups orzo

4 cups chicken stock

½ cup natural plain yoghurt

2 tbsp tomato paste

3 oz/150g fresh spinach

1 tbsp fresh rosemary or thyme, finely chopped

2 tbsp fresh parsley, finely chopped

Zest of 1 lemon

2 tbsp parmesan, finely grated

1 tsp chilli flakes (optional)

Method

1. For the meatballs, preheat the oven to 350F/180C. Prepare a baking tray with some baking parchment paper.

2. In a mixing bowl add your ground chicken, breadcrumbs, granulated garlic, rosemary, chilli flakes, parsley, sundried tomatoes, salt and pepper. Mix everything well together.

3. Form 12-16 meatballs (depending on the size of your balls). Place them on your prepared baking tray, brush each one with a little olive oil and bake for 25-30 minutes until gorgeous and golden.

4. For the orzo get your saucepan on a medium to low heat. Add 1tbsp olive oil, shallots, garlic, chilli flakes and season with a pinch of salt. Gentle cook for 2-3 minutes.

5. Stir your tomato paste cook for another minute. Add 1 cup of your chicken stock, then add your orzo, bring to a simmer and cook for 2 minutes. Add the rest of your chicken stock and cook

for a further 6 minutes, stirring often.

6. Add your spinach to the orzo and continue cooking until the spinach has wilted. Take off the heat and add your yogurt, parsley and lemon zest. Taste and season with salt and pepper.

7. Serve your chicken meatballs over your orzo, sprinkle your parmesan over your meatball and enjoy this delicious dish! xX

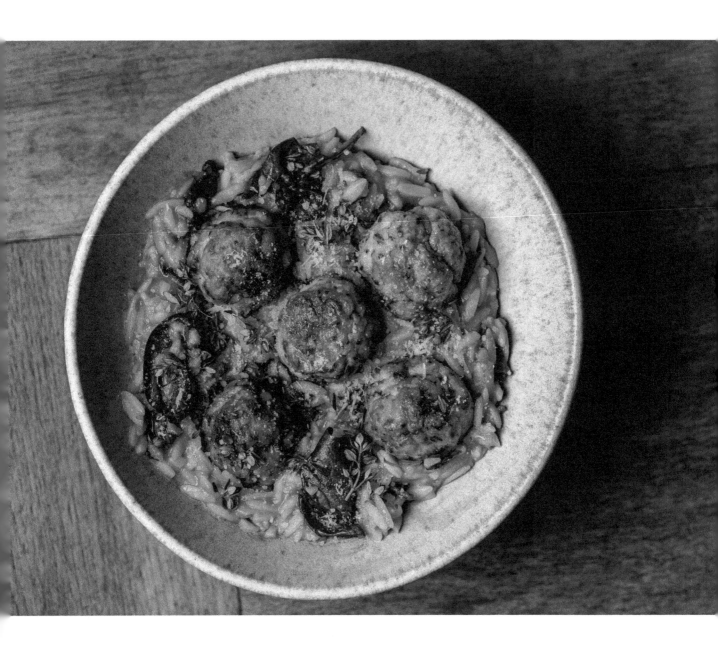

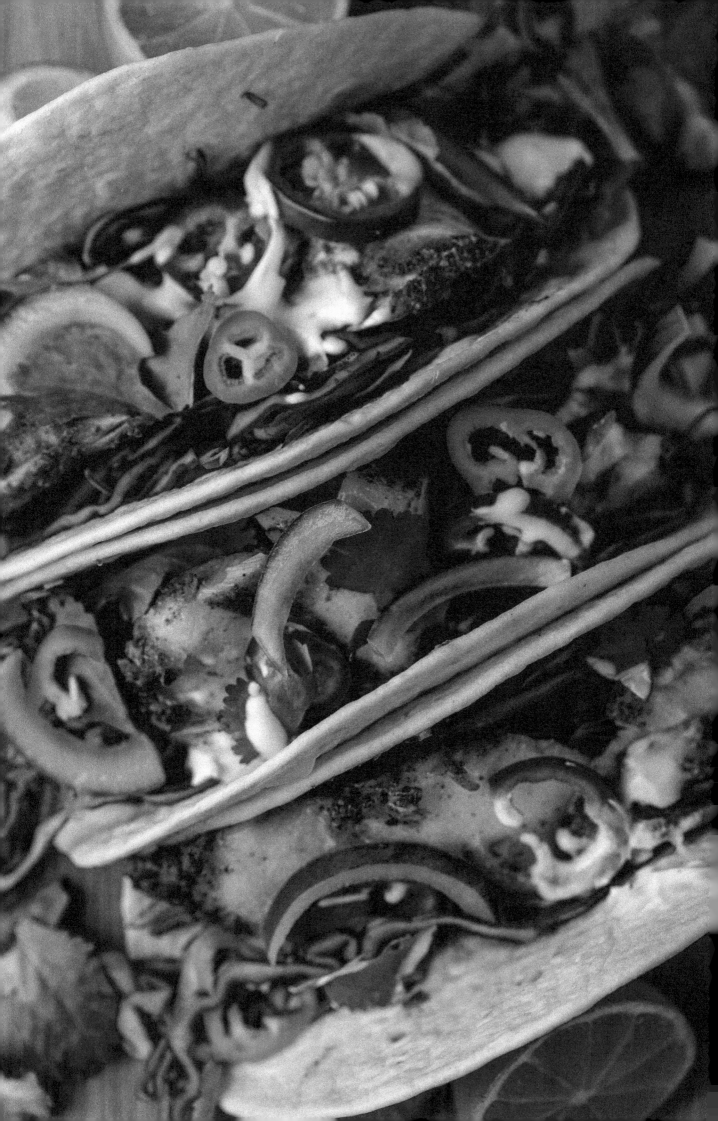

Blackened Fish Tacos

exican food is an absolute favourite of ours! That's why we wanted to create a healthy fish taco, which was simple to cook but packed full of flavour. Wherever we have been in the world together there is always fresh fish, with tropical zinging flavours involved. Lots of chatting, usually about our questionable love lives and always with a cheeky margarita on the rocks! We cannot get enough of these fish tacos; you are going to love them too!

Ingredients

Serves 4

4 fillets/24 ounces of firm white fish like cod or mahi mahi

4 tbsp Cajian spice mix

½ small red cabbage, shredded

4 limes

1 jar of jalapenos

2 small avocados

1 small red onion, finely chopped

2 tomatoes, chopped

1 red pepper, finely chopped

1 bunch fresh coriander, roughly chopped

1 mango, diced (optional)

12 corn tortillas

Olive oil

Salt and pepper

Method

1. Pre heat the oven to 350F/180C. Cut your fish into thick finger slices drizzle with some olive oil rub all over the fish, then coat the fish with the Cajian spice so the fish fingers are evenly covered all over.

2. Place the fish on a lined baking tray and put in the oven. Cook for 10-12 minutes until the fish is cooked through and flaky.

3. Make the guacamole by mashing up the avocado in a bowl with a fork, season with salt and pepper and the juice of 1 lime, add your red onion, red pepper and tomato. Give the guacamole a good mix taste, drizzle with a little olive oil and add a little more salt and pepper if needed.

4. In a small blender add half a bunch of coriander, 2tbsp jalapeños, juice of 1 lime, 2tbsp olive oil and salt and pepper. Roughly blend and you have a simple spicy salsa to go over your tacos for a little more flavour.

5. Start to build your tacos by putting your red cabbage, followed by flaking the fish on top, then good dollops of your guacamole, chopped mango (if using), sliced jalapeno, coriander then a squeeze of lime and your cilantro and jalapeno salsa drizzled over the top! They are now ready to be demolished!

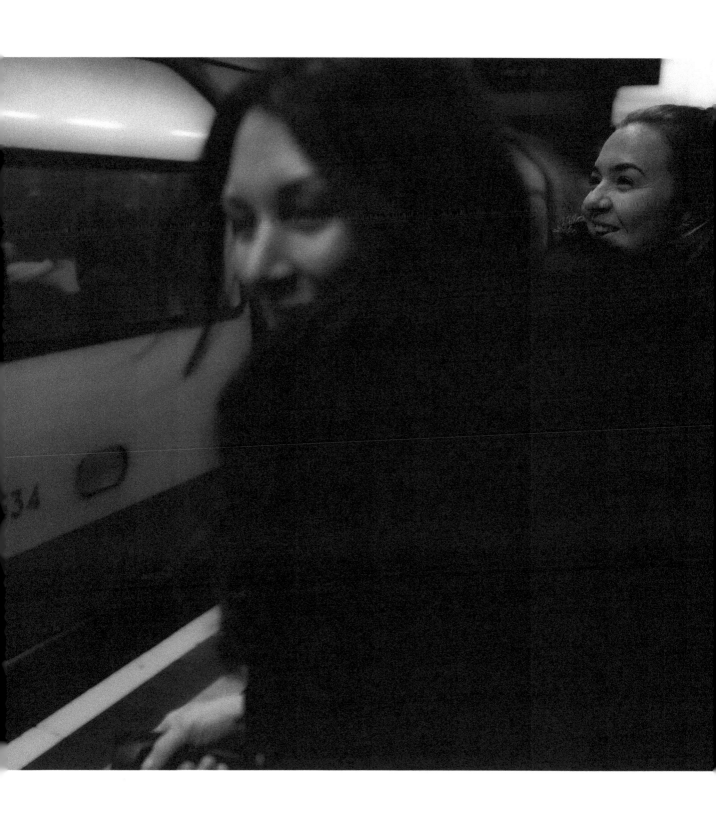

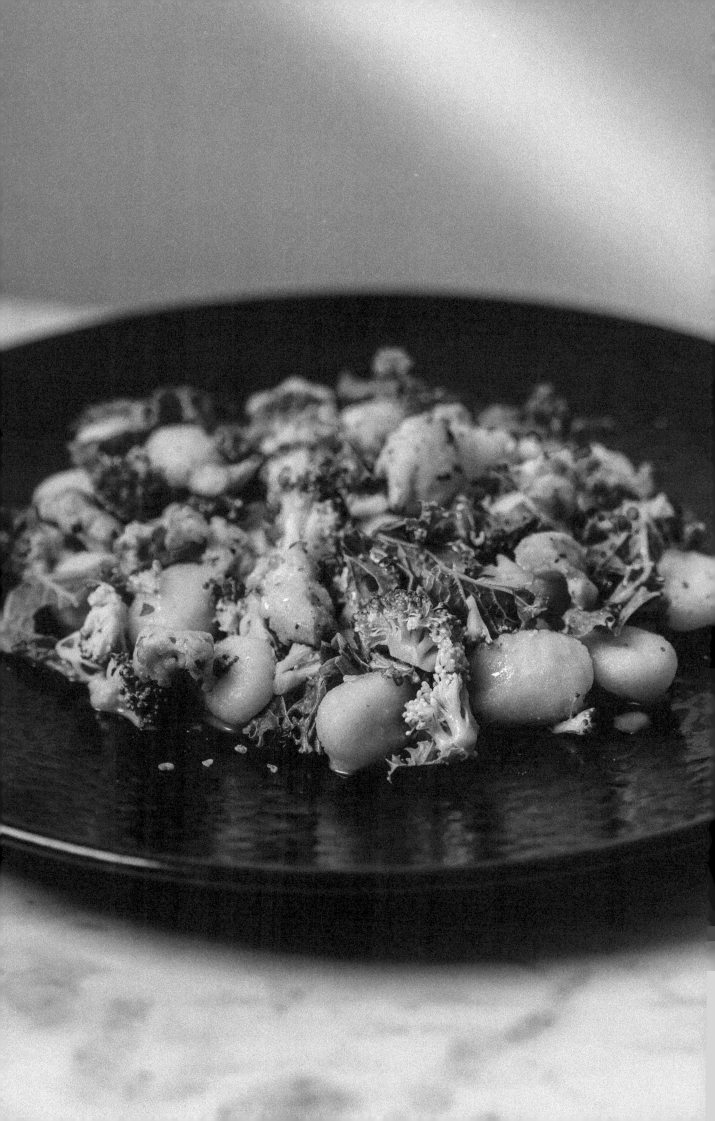

Broccoli Kale Sausage Pesto Gnocchi

This dish is so delicious and with a silky pesto sauce without adding any cream, just more protein with the egg yolk! We can chow down to this anytime of the year! You can switch up the pasta to any kind you like and if you want to be a little more indulgent swap the chicken sausage for pork. Enjoy hunnies

Ingredients
Serves 2

4 chicken sausages, skin removed, and meat broken into pieces

12oz / 350g gnocchi

3oz / 90g kale, stakes removed and roughly chopped

7oz / 200g tenderstem broccoli, cut into 3rds

2oz / 50g parmesan cheese, finely grated

2 tbsp pesto

1 tsp chili flakes optional

1 tsp fennel seed optional

Zest of 1 lemon

1 egg yolk

Olive oil

Salt and pepper

Method

1. Put your egg yolk in a cup add half of your parmesan to the egg yolk, with the lemon zest, chilli flakes, pesto and a good pinch of salt and pepper. Give it a good mix. Set aside as you are going

to add 4 tbsp of the starchy water the gnocchi will be cooked in before you drain the pasta.

2. In a frying pan add 1 tbsp of oil, bring the pan to a medium heat add your chicken sausage and fennel if using. Cook until the chicken is nicely browned on the outside and cooked through on the inside.

3. Bring a pan of water to the boil (life hack boil the kettle and pour into a pan). Add your gnocchi and tenderstem broccoli cook for 3 mins, add your kale after 2 minutes. Before you drain add 4 tbsp of the pasta water to your egg yolk mixture.

4. Drain the pasta, add the egg yolk mixture to your empty pasta pan, add your gnocchi, broccoli and kale back to the pan with your egg yolk mixture, then add your chicken sausage and bring back to a very low heat. Coat the gnocchi, sausage and veggies with the mixture until it becomes silky this will only take around two minutes.

5. Now get this creamy sausage, veggie gnocchi into your bowls, sprinkle with the rest of your parmesan and freshly ground pepper. Enjoy this delicious dish with a healthy twist!

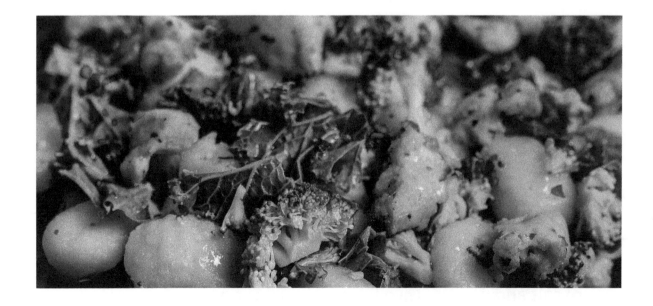

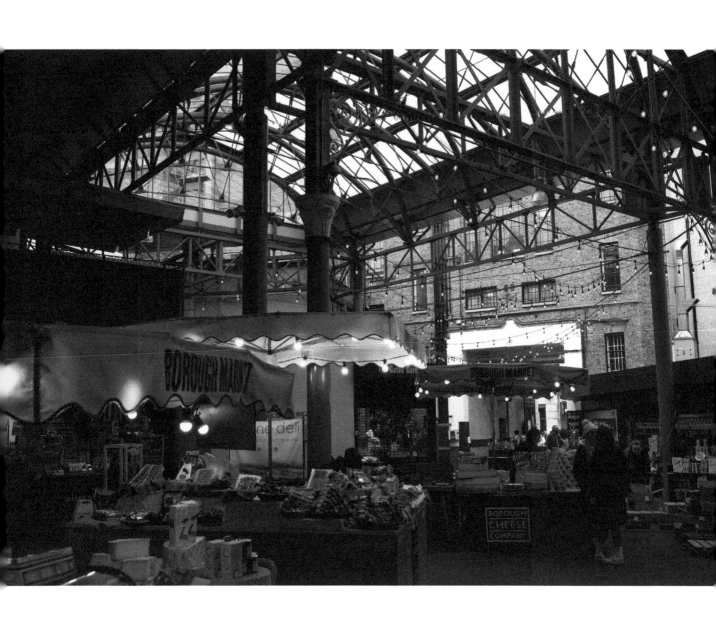

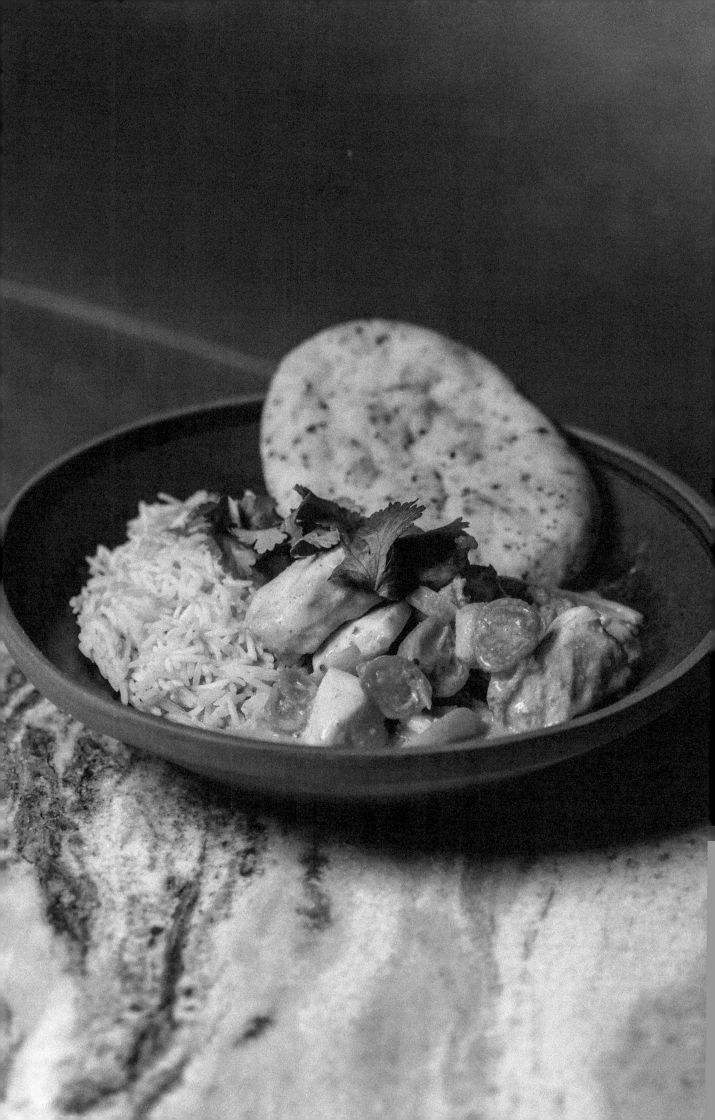

Easy Healthy Fish Curry

ish curry is one of our favourite dishes! When we are in Antigua together one of our favourite places is a little Indian restaurant called Indian summer, which overlooks Falmouth marina. They do the best Indian food and this is a take on one of their amazing fish curries! We also used to grab a takeaway from there and take it up to Shirley's heights and watch the sunset putting the world to rights over a bottle of Rose!

Ingredients
Serves 4

1 lb 12oz / 800g skinless firm white fish, cut into large chunks

½ tsp hot chilli powder

1 tsp ground turmeric

2-3 green chillies, roughly chopped

2 onions, finely slice

A thumb size piece of ginger, finely chopped

2 cloves of garlic, finely chopped

1 tbsp mustard seeds

1 can / 14oz vine tomatoes, roughly chopped

1 can / 14oz tin coconut milk

150ml / 5oz chicken, fish or veggie stock

2 tbsp tamarind paste

1 tbsp honey

Salt and pepper

Small bunch fresh cilantro / coriander

1 lime, juiced

Olive oil

Rice to serve

Method

1. Mix the lime juice, turmeric and chilli powder in a large bowl with a pinch of salt. Add the fish pieces and carefully toss in the marinade.

2. Heat a little oil in a large wide pan, or deep frying pan and fry the sliced onions on a medium to low heat for 6 minutes with a pinch of salt. Add the garlic, ginger, green chilli and mustard seeds, cook for another 3 minutes.

3. Now add the tomatoes and stock. Fry for 5 minutes. Then add the coconut milk. Simmer for 10 minutes until thickened slightly. Season, add the tamarind paste and honey.

4. Now add the fish mixture and gently tuck them into the sauce and poach the fish for 5 minutes until the fish is cooked through and has started to flake.

Serve with some lovely fluffy rice and finish off with fresh coriander. Enjoy this delicious fish of healthy yumminess! xX

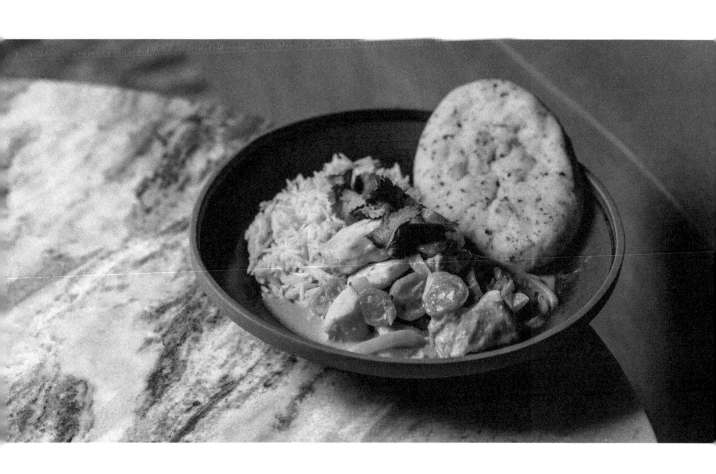

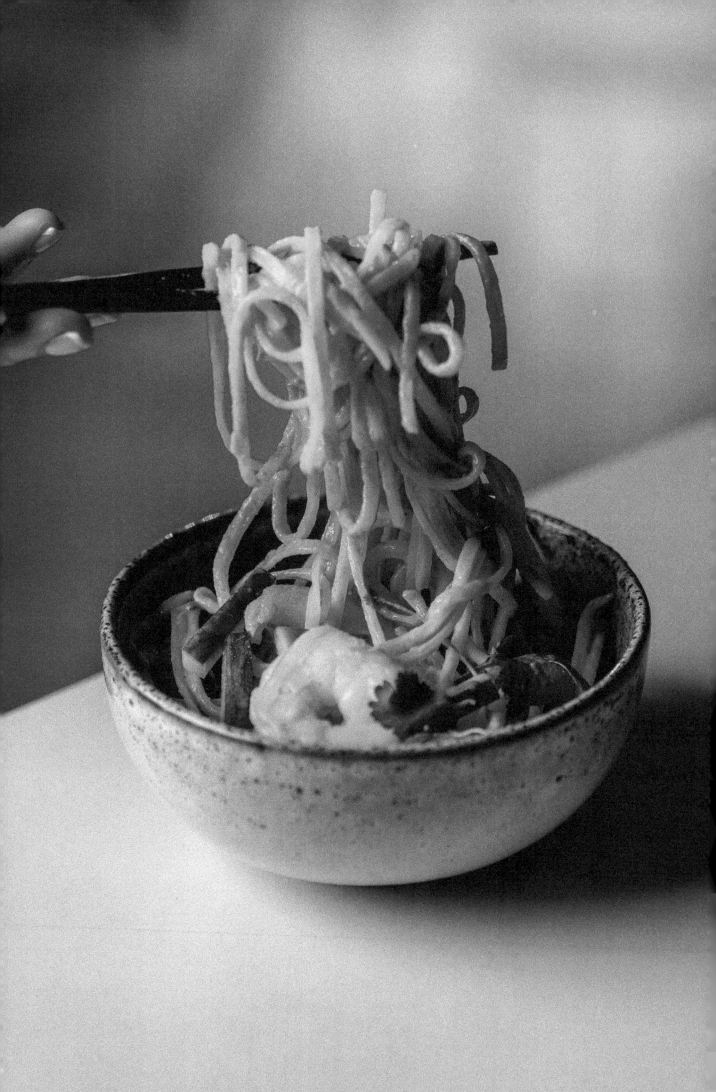

Easy Prawn Laksa

This dish is simply delish!!! You never want to do a recipe when you need 101 ingredients because, 'Ain't nobody got time for that'. But you also want something tasty, simple and healthy. We are obsessed with this dish; if prawns aren't your thing, you can use chicken, tofu or beef. Run, don't walk to cook this one!

Ingredients
Serves 2

100g / 3.5oz medium rice noodles

2 tbsp peanut butter or almond butter

1 cans / 14oz of ½ fat coconut milk

500ml / 16oz chicken or vegan stock

300g / 10oz of large prawns or tofu

1 tsp turmeric

2 tbsp Thai red curry paste

1 lime, juiced

2 tbsp honey or agave

2 large handfuls of beansprouts

1/4 cucumber, seeds removed and cut into strips

Small bunch fresh coriander

1 red chilli, deseeded and finely sliced (optional)

Method

1. Cook the noodles as per the packet instructions. Set aside.

2. In a small blender blend the Thai red curry paste, nut butter,

turmeric, honey/agave, lime juice and 1 of the red chillies, if you like it nice and spicy! Blend and if it needs some liquid to loosen the paste, add a bit of your stock.

3. Add the blended paste to your pan and cook on a medium to low heat, then add the coconut milk and stock, stir and cook on a medium heat for 4-5 minutes. Add your prawns and cook through until they turn pink.

4. Get your serving bowls ready. Before you add the noodles to your bowls run the noodles briefly under cold water, as this will loosen them so they won't stick together while you are trying to divide them up. Ladle your laksa and prawns into your bowls. Top with beansprouts, matchstick cucumber, coriander and chilli, sit down and start sluuurping!

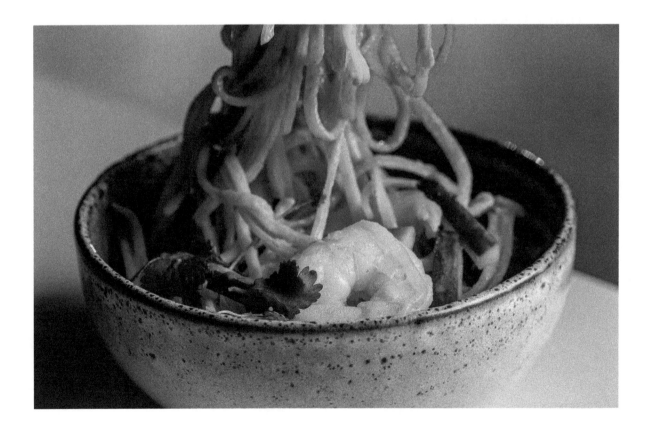

Bryony Johnson & Daisy Kellihe

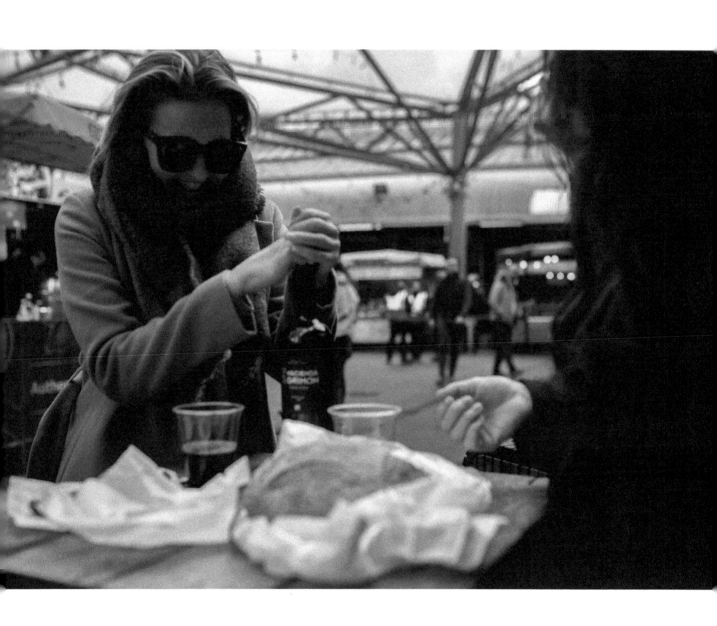

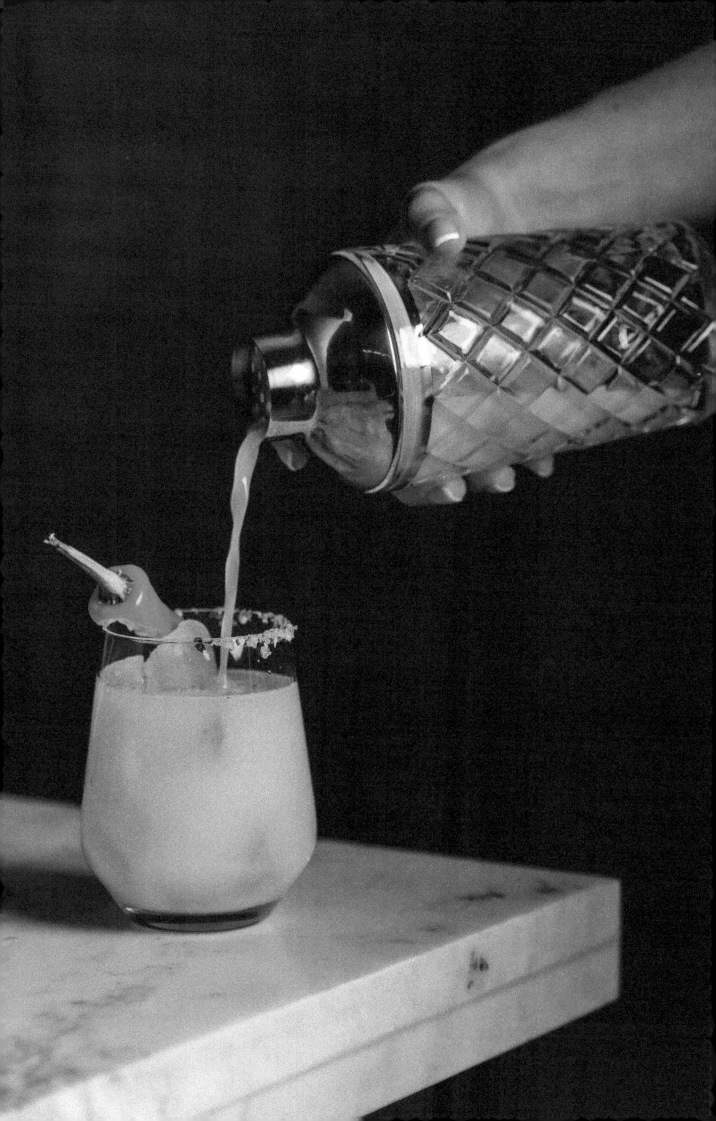

Daisy's Margarita

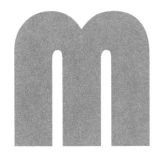argaritas are one of our all-time favourite cocktails. We have shared so many good memories and set the world straight sharing copious amounts of these delicious drinks together. Shock horror, that Daisy was not originally a fan of tequila but that all changed when she started working on a boat for a Texan family, who had such a strong love for Mexico. They taught Daisy the recipe, and she did not dare change it! That same recipe has gone all over the world with Daisy and to say it gets the party started is an understatement. We hope it brings you as many happy memories with your friends and family as it has with ours!

Ingredients

Makes 1 amazing marg!

40ml / 1 ½ oz of silver tequila

40ml / 1 ½ oz of triple sec (a dash extra if you like it sweeter)

40ml / 1 ½ oz freshly squeezed lime juice

Method

1. Coat the rim of the margarita glass with lime juice then dip the rim in salt and chilli flakes, or half the rim if you are like me.

2. Pour the ingredients into a cocktail shaker. Give it a good little shake.

3. Pour the mix over ice into your margarita glass. Chin Chin!!!

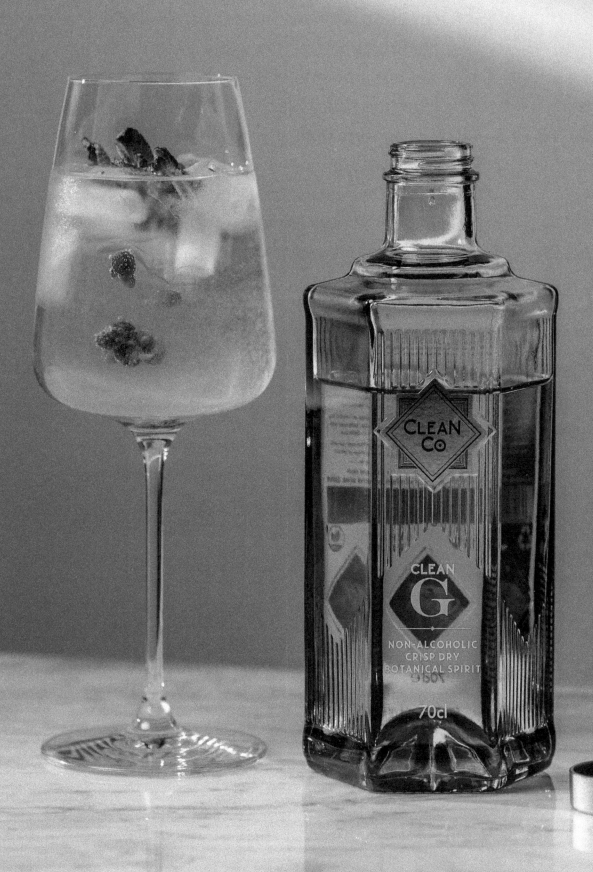

Pom Pom Gin

for us, this drink is a reminder of perfect spring/summer days, where we drank a few of these together when we were both in London. When the sun shines and summer starts to make an appearance, it's time to pull out the gin, make this refreshing drink, sit in the garden, take a sip and begin to imagine all the possibilities that summer may bring. Enjoy this cocktail and think of the endless warm nights and what they have in store for you...

Ingredients
Makes 1 drink

1 small handful of fresh raspberries

1 tbsp fresh pomegranate seeds

40ml / 1 ½ oz gin

½ lime, juice

Handful of fresh mint leaves

1 can of tonic or soda water which ever you prefer

Method

1. Squash your raspberries and pomegranates together.

2. Strain through a sieve into a gin glass

3. Add your lime juice.

4. Pour your gin and top your glass with your tonic or soda water and garnish with some fresh mint leaves!

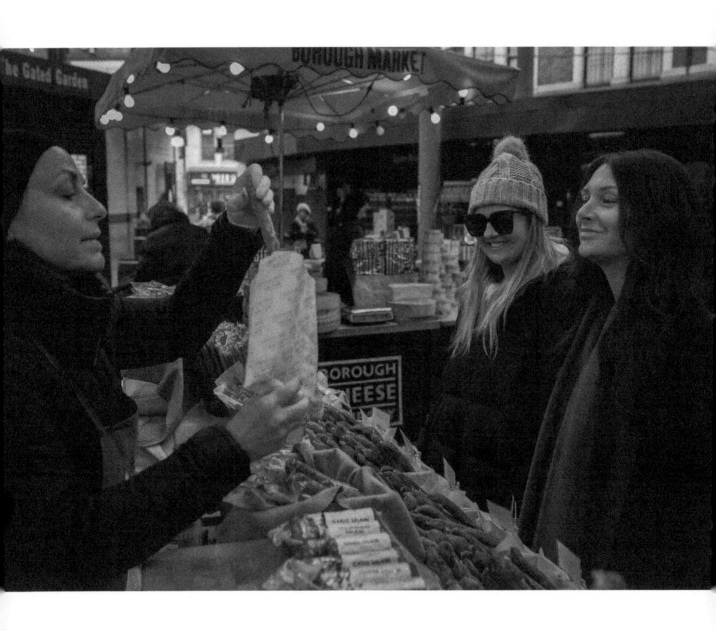

Thank you...

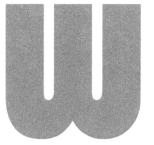

We would like to take this opportunity to say thank you to the people who were able to make this book possible;

Emma Pharaoh did our food photography. She was incredible, gave us so much direction and made the whole day so enjoyable. We love the photos. As you can see, she did an incredible job.

Instagram - emmapharaohphoto

Tom Silcock, who did our photos for our day out in London. We came up with the concept together, we wanted the book to show our daily lives in the city and the activities we enjoy together. Tom is a good friend and he made us feel so at ease. We loved the whole day and the images captured depicts exactly the fun we had!

Instagram - tms_slk

Anna Glynn, a great friend, is responsible for getting our front cover which we also love! We literally did this off an iphone and were delighted with the photo, so a big thank you to Anna for taking time out of her day to take this.

Rick Armstrong and **Rich Hayden** from **Fisher King Publishing**, are the team responsible for putting the book together, without their patience and guidance Galley Girls would have never come to life!

The amazing traders of Borough Market. If you are in London and looking for amazing produce, you must get along to Borough Market; it has an incredible vibe and is well worth a visit. We loved our day there. Everyone we met was incredible, we owe you all a huge thank you. They were so informative, helpful and friendly and we left with the most amazing products and produce.

Our dinner photos were taken in **Los Mochis in Notting Hill**. This is the place where we came up with the Galley Girls concept so it is fitting that we give this restaurant a special mention. If you are in the area we highly recommend booking a table at Los Mochis.

We have teamed up with **Savernake Knives**, which we are beyond excited about. We were invited to the factory where we were shown around, brainstormed and came up with our bespoke knives. We are delighted to be working with them and love our knives so much. Thank you Savernake Knives, you are incredible!

Instagram - savernake_knives

Finally, but not least, we would like to thank **Justine Murphy** at **MyMuyBueno** for kindly letting us use her kitchen to prepare the meals for the photos.

Instagram - mymuybueno

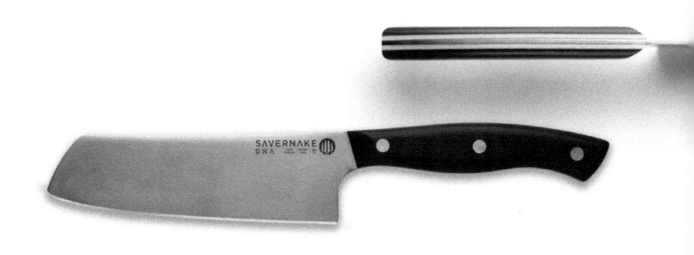